Subtle
Aromatherapy

D0769866

By the same author:

Aromatherapy: An A–Z
A Change for the Better

SUBTLE AROMATHERAPY

Patricia Davis

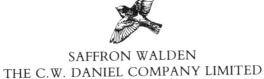

SAFFRON WALDEN
THE C.W. DANIEL COMPANY LIMITED

First published in Great Britain in 1991
by The C.W. Daniel Company Limited,
1, Church Path, Saffron Walden,
Essex. CB10 1JP, England

© Patricia Davis 1991

ISBN 0 85207 227 9

Reprinted December 1992
Reprinted May 1996

Designed by Dale Dawson
Production in association with
Book Production Consultants, Cambridge
Typeset by Cambridge Photosetting Services
Printed and bound by St Edmundsbury Press, Bury St Edmunds, Suffolk.

Dedication

This book is dedicated to Marie, who opened the door.

Acknowledgements

I offer my sincere thanks to Caroline Wyndham and Simon Alleguen for their valuable collaboration on the Crystals chapter; to Marie Herbert for commenting on 'Sex, Spirit and Essential Oils' from her rich experience as a psychosynthesis counsellor; to Claire Harvey for insights into flower essences; to Andy Ellis for material on geopathic stress; to David Cousins and Richard Offut for healing and guidance; to my many colleagues and friends for sharing their professional experience; to my son, Ben Shallcross for steering me through the minefields of word-processing and above all to my unseen guides for the channelled information I have received while writing this book.

Contents

Preface

The information that I have gathered together in this book has come to me in many different ways: through my personal experience as an aromatherapist and user of essential oils in my everyday life; through the shared experiences of my colleagues and friends; from voracious reading about other ways of using plant energies; from my lifelong interest in myths, fairytales, folklore and anthropology; from my personal experience of meditation and from deeply-felt intuition. Some of the information in this book is directly channelled, so that at the end of writing I know more than I did at the beginning, and for this gift I am profoundly grateful.

Above all, the oils have been my teachers. Much of what you will find written here I have learnt from directly working with essential oils. Always, when writing about a particular oil, I have had that oil beside me on the desk, smelt it, poured out a drop and looked at it, allowing myself to be receptive to everything that the colour, texture, smell and 'personality' of that oil could tell me. Sometimes I have been surprised: what I discovered about the subtle properties of that oil was not always what I expected.

I earnestly suggest that you do the same. Approach the oils with sensitivity and an open mind and see what they can tell you about themselves. Your experience may not be the same as mine, and neither your experience nor mine will necessarily be the same at different times. So, please use this book as a general guide, and as a starting point for your own exploration.

Some of this information you can find for yourself in a

variety of places, but I believe this is the first time it has been gathered together in one book. There is also much that has not been set down in writing before. Apart from knowledge channelled through me during the writing of this book, there is information I have previously shared only with trusted colleagues, for fear that it might be misused. But there is a greater need for subtle therapies now than ever before. There is a spiritual awakening abroad on our planet, and an urgent feeling among those who hold esoteric knowledge that it must be shared with all who genuinely seek it.

I believe that Subtle Aromatherapy is one of the many avenues open to us for personal and spiritual growth, as well as for helping our clients and friends towards physical, mental and spiritual wholeness, so I have set out here everything that I have been able to learn in this field. I do not put myself forward as an expert: I still have much to learn but I feel that what I do know must be shared.

> *May all Beings be well.*
> *May all Beings be happy.*
> *May all Beings live in Peace.*

Totnes,
Devon,
Midsummer Day, 1991

CHAPTER 1

What is Subtle Aromatherapy?

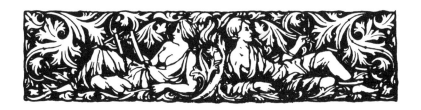

What is Subtle Aromatherapy? In using this expression I have in mind primarily the use of essential oils in non-physical ways. Subtle Aromatherapy makes use of the oils to affect the subtle body, the psyche and, indeed, the soul. In doing so, the user draws on the subtle, energetic or vibrational qualities of essential oils, rather than their physical properties. The expression can be used to denote the use of essential oils to heal the physical body by influencing the subtle or energetic body of the recipient so Subtle Aromatherapy may be described as one form of vibrational healing. It also embraces the use of essential oils as an aid to meditation, affirmations, visualization and all transformative techniques based on inner work.

Because of the versatility of essential oils, they can be used in many different ways. When they are used with massage to treat a variety of physical ills (and this is the most important method of application in what I shall call 'traditional' aromatherapy) they act on the body in a very gentle, though effective way. This, though, is still a physical therapy and as such is not the main focus of this book, even though it is true that a physical aromatherapy massage can often have profound and beneficial effects on a less tangible level. Most clients report a feeling of uplift or release of anxiety after such treatment but that is still not Subtle Aromatherapy.

In Subtle Aromatherapy the therapist may not touch the client's body at all, or may incorporate elements of subtle aromatherapy into a hand-on treatment. In some instances there may be no need for a therapist, as in the use of aromatics in burners or diffusers as a meditation aid, or in ritual bathing.

Some applications of essential oils that can be properly described as Subtle Aromatherapy are auric massage, chakra balancing, absent healing, planetary healing, meditation, ritual and religious ceremony, and the use of oils to help personal growth on both the personality and the spiritual level. These are by no means all the possibilities: you may well find yourself guided towards others of which I am not yet aware. There are no 'right' or 'wrong' ways of working in Subtle Aromatherapy. Provided you act with honesty and sensitivity, whichever way you work is right.

In the past decade traditional aromatherapy has been more widely practised, studied and described than ever before. Thanks to recent and ongoing research we now have a wealth of knowledge about the physical properties and actions of essential oils: their chemical make-up, their action against specific bacteria and viruses, why certain oils are hazardous, how they enter the bloodstream, how they affect the various organs of the body, the mechanics of olfaction and even a little about how they affect the brain. New oils are being discovered and introduced, as well as different varieties of the oils we already know. More books are being written, more teachers are travelling around the world sharing their knowledge. This does not necessarily make us into better aromatherapists than our predecessors who based their judgement to a large extent on the accumulated experience of centuries. It does make us better-informed aromatherapists, maybe more 'scientific' aromatherapists, though whether or not that is a good thing is the subject of much discussion and some disagreement.

Parallel with this increasing volume of factual information about physical aromatherapy has been a growing desire to know more about the non-physical effects of essential oils. The action of essential oils on the mind is, of course, far harder to study and far more open to differing interpretation than their physical action. We know a very little about how the physical structures of the brain receive and interpret information from the olfactory cells, and even something about how brain activity changes when essential oils are inhaled. But the brain is not the mind and no amount of physical investigation can tell us how the mind works, let alone how essential oils affect it. The study of psychology can help us to understand something of the workings of the mind, but for any knowledge of how essentials oils interact with the human mind, we cannot study the workings, we can only observe the effects. This may be through using an oil personally and noticing the effect it has on our mood, mental state or emotions, by noting and recording how our clients feel after using various oils, by exchanging information with other therapists in person or reading about their experiences and – just as with the physical effects of oils – by drawing on the wealth of experience that has been recorded since written records of essential oils, herbs and other aromatics began.

Traditional knowledge is the basis on which all modern practice is founded and should never be lightly dismissed. For example, where a modern textbook describes an oil as antidepressant and we find an old herbal stating that the plant from which it is distilled 'maketh glad the heart' they are saying exactly the same thing in the differing terminology of their respective historical periods.

When we wish to study the most subtle effects of essential oils, we have even less to go on. If the study of mind is fraught with difficulty, the study of the subtle body and the soul or, if you prefer, the higher self or human spirituality, is even more so and if you wish to learn about the subtle or spiritual connotations of essential oils and plants you will find little in the existing aromatherapy literature to help. You will need to explore the holy books of the various religions, the writing of mystics, alchemists and astrologers, myth and legend, folklore, fairytales, fables and even old wives' tales for references to sacred plants, incenses, anointing oils, 'magical' potions and elixirs and herbal talismans. You will also need to sift through the nonsense and the work of charlatans that can get mixed up in some of these sources, as well as discarding references to essential oils that we know to be hazardous (remember that earlier usage probably referred to the fresh or dried plant which may be safer to handle). The knowledge of earlier civilisations can be very enriching, as can that of so-called 'primitive' civilisations who are often closer to the earth and its plants in both their mundane and spiritual lives than we moderns.

None of these sources, though, can take the place of personal experience. Experiencing essential oils as an aid to one's own personal growth or spiritual development, or to bring about healing without 'hands on' treatment is the surest way to learn what effects they have. Next best is hearing of the experiences of other aromatherapists who have used oils in these ways and at present such individual exchange is the principle way in which knowledge of the subtle or spiritual properties of essential oils is spread, since little has been written about them.

Although most training courses in traditional aromatherapy include some work on essential oils and the mind, few teachers offer guidance on subtle uses when training future therapists. Perhaps this is just as well, for I think it is good to have a solid understanding of traditional aromatherapy before experimenting with the more esoteric uses of essential oils.

Of course, it is impossible to draw a clear line between traditional aromatherapy and subtle uses of essential oils and some therapists have discovered these uses for themselves by 'accident'. This often happens when both the therapist and the person receiving treatment are spiritually aware, maybe regular meditators, psychic, or attuned to subtle energies in one way or another. A massage session planned to affect the physical body and perhaps the mental/ emotional level may then take on another dimension. The client may report seeing colours or light, or feeling a sensation of floating, as though the massage couch had been removed. These are the experiences most commonly reported, though a small number of people have described past-life recall, out-of-body states, vivid visual impressions or a mental state akin to deep meditation. Such experiences often leave the individual with feelings of deep bliss.

In my own work, and as a recipient of aromatherapy massage, I have either experienced or witnessed all of these. I consider such experiences very important, because they were not anticipated and this refutes the sceptic's claim that 'You only felt that because that is what you expected to feel'.

Such experiences often serve as a starting point from which an individual begins to explore other possibilities in the use of essential oils. They may be guided by drawing analogies with the physical or mental effects of the oils, and such analogies are valuable indications of what an oil may do when used in more subtle ways.

However, as we enter the dawn of a new age, an increasing number of people feel drawn to using essential oils at subtle levels who have not been through the traditional 'apprenticeship' of learning to use essential oils in physical applications first so they do not have that basis from which to start working. Such people include healers, crystal workers, meditators, clairvoyants and others. They may have had some experience of essential oils being used in a meditation group, at a meeting or workshop or read something about them that has aroused their interest and suggested possible areas of affinity with their own field of interest.

Others, who do have experience of the physical applications of essential oils, feel a need to move on from this base. As a greater awareness of our spiritual destiny is awakened in the world, many people practising physical therapies feel drawn to working in a less physical way. They may wish to incorporate a spiritual or subtle element into the work they are doing already, or they may eventually want to change their mode of working completely.

To everyone who would like to explore the subtle uses of essential oils, I extend an invitation to share my journey of discovery.

CHAPTER 2

Vibrational Healing

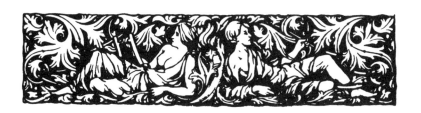

Nothing in the universe is still.

G reat stars pulsate, their planets circle round them, clouds of gases swirl around, stars explode into life or crumble into death. On our own planet Earth it is easy to observe the constant movement of the winds and oceans, less easy to comprehend the movement of great mountain ranges. But the Earth herself is constantly moving. As well as her endless circle dance through space, she moves within herself. Continents shift, slowly but inexorably, hot springs bubble out from Earth's crust, lava flows. Sometimes the movement is violent and we call it an earthquake, but even at times of the greatest stillness every particle of Earth's substance is moving. The greatest mountains, the most immovable rocks are moving within each of their atoms.

The dance of the atom reflects the dance of the solar system, for every particle within an atom spins around the neutron – the atom's Sun. None of this movement is random; the pattern of movement within each atom is as organised and inexorable as the movement of planets in their orbits.

When we look at living organisms that same pattern becomes apparent. Within the human body, for example, the heart pulses blood through the veins, lymph courses along its own channels, air flows into and out of the lungs, minute electrical impulses speed along nerve pathways to and from the brain. Even when the body is completely still, the heart still beats and the lungs empty and fill without our volition.

If we look at the body in the most minute detail every one of its millions of cells vibrates with its own life pattern; each minute component of the cell dancing round its nucleus. The inner dance of the cells is no more random than the inner dance of the atom. Just as every atom of Oxygen, for example, dances to the same rhythm as every other atom of

Oxygen, which is different from that of an atom of Gold or an atom of Nitrogen, so the cells of the brain execute their own dance, which is not the same as the dance of the heart's cells.

Every cell in the human body is born knowing its own dance, the pattern that was ordained for that cell even before the moment of conception and which every cell carries encoded in its genetic material to be passed on to new cells as they, in turn, are born.

As science finds ever more powerful ways of making the invisible visible, we can see the exquisite harmony of the movement of cells. Photographed through an electron microscope, for example, the cells' dance manifests as beautiful and symmetrical patterns. This harmony is both a reflection of the cell's health and the source of that health, for as long as the cell moves in its ordered dance every function of that cell will take place in an orderly way, and we experience this as the state of health. If the order breaks down, and the movements within the cell become random, or different from their pre-ordained pattern, then the function of the cell is disturbed, too, and dis-ease will follow. This too can be seen in micro-photographs: the pattern of dis-eased cells is distorted, it does not have the beauty and symmetry that we associate with healthy cells.

On these facts all systems of vibrational medicine are based.

Surgery and cytotoxic drugs aim to remove or kill the diseased cells. Techniques such as ultra-sound or radiotherapy impose their own pattern of vibration on the cells as a means of changing a dis-eased pattern of movement into a harmonious one. Medicinal drugs, whether synthetic or naturally-occurring, influence the vibration of cells by physically introducing new elements and therefore new vibrations into the cell's structure.

But Subtle Aromatherapy and all the various systems or therapies which may be described as vibrational healing aim to restore harmony by subtle means, by using what we might think of as gentle persuasion to nudge discordant, and therefore dis-eased, cells back into their original pattern of vibration, thereby restoring health.

I would like you to imagine a large ballroom, with hundreds of couples dancing to a lyrical waltz. Each couple rotates smoothly on its own axis, as well as progressing round the room in the same direction as all the other couples. All move to the same rhythm, maintained by the orchestra, and we can reasonably assume that everybody is happy and relaxed. Suddenly, an intruder bursts into the ballroom and grabs hold of one couple with angry words and gestures. Other dancers swerve to avoid the argument, but in doing so they bump into each other and come to a halt. Perhaps they react angrily to this disruption of their enjoyment, and a group of angry, shouting, gesticulating people quickly surround the intruder. The noise increases until nobody can hear the music at all and the dancing comes to a halt. Maybe by now fists are flying and some-body has been hurt. But now the bouncers are on the scene and, grabbing the intruder, they forcibly try to get him out of the ballroom. He resists, of course, flailing and shouting. He may get hurt, the bouncers may get hurt, possibly some of the bystanders, too, but eventually he is pushed out into the night and peace is restored. Maybe the dance will resume, but maybe by now everybody is so upset that they don't feel like dancing anymore, and the orchestra leader decides to pack up and go home.

But now imagine, if you will, that among those present there is somebody of a very calm disposition, but powerful personality, who quickly spots the initial disturbance, speaks quietly but convincingly to the intruder and persuades him to step aside and discuss his grievances. Very few of the other dancers realise that anything unusual has happened at all. Only those nearest the scene know that anything was

13

wrong, and they are soon able to resume their stately dance. The orchestra continues to play, the music can be heard by everybody and the ball continues uninterrupted until the dancers are ready to go home, tired but happy.

Of course, that would be a happier solution, but perhaps it would have been even better if a perceptive friend had noticed the potential intruder's distress and taken steps to make him feel happier and calmer before the night of the ball. Then no disturbance would have taken place at all.

You might like to think of this little scenario as a metaphor for dis-ease and the various ways in which we attempt to heal it. It cannot be denied that the bouncers do an efficient job, but many of us would prefer to see the intruder persuaded to leave by gentler means or, better still, helped in some way before any trouble arose.

Vibrational healing takes account of the fact that disturbed vibrations arise in the subtle body before disease manifests on the physical plane, often a long time before. To gently help restore these vibrations to their original state of harmony before physical dis-ease occurs is surely better than waiting until drugs, surgery or other invasive means are needed to correct it. Even when physical disease has developed, it may be reversed by changing the subtle energy. I'm sure you have read of cases where cancers have disappeared after the patient practised healing visualization techniques, or of apparently 'hopeless cases' cured by healers after orthodox medicine had given up.

It is also important to realise that disturbed vibrations can stay within the subtle body after physical healing appears to have taken place. Slow recovery, relapse and failure to heal fully can all be due to this phenomenon, so it is wise to seek out a therapist who practises one or other of the subtle therapies as soon as possible after surgery, road accidents, falls or any other events that may upset the delicate balance that exists between the subtle and physical bodies.

Before exploring some of the techniques that can be described as vibrational healing I would like to look at the idea of vibration itself. All vibration is movement but not all movement is vibration. Movement such as walking, dancing, digging the garden are not vibration, nor is mechanical movement such as rocks rolling down a hillside, or a car speeding down the motorway.

Vibration could be defined as a continuous series of minute movements, repeated without variation. If the movement does vary, it becomes a different vibration altogether.

We are surrounded by vibration at all times. Our perception of the outer world depends on it, and our sensory organs – ears, eyes, nose – are in fact finely tuned receptors for various kinds of vibration. Our eyes detect all the various vibrations of light that appear to us as colour, our ears receive sound vibrations, and it has only recently been shown that our noses, too, detect smell in much the same way, by responding to the vibrations of different aromatic molecules.

Many analogies can be made between colour, sound and smell. We speak of sounds being high or low, harmonious or discordant. A visual artist will use the same terms to describe colours and combinations of colour. Perfumiers and aromatherapists borrow the musical language to describe aromas (which are very hard to describe in words). We talk of an essential oil having a high or low 'note' and this was elaborated about a hundred years ago into an elegant theory of Top, Middle and Base notes when a perfumier called Piesse arranged odours on a stave, exactly like a musical scale. We also use the painter's vocabulary to describe aromas, using words like 'a green scent' or the 'highlight' of a perfume. We blend several oils to make a new aroma, just as the painter blends various pigments to make a different colour.

These analogies are of use to the therapist both in

relating the treatment to the vibrational needs of the client, and in combining two or more therapies. For example, an increasing number of people now use colour therapy and aromatherapy together, and they find analogies between colours and aromas often suggest themselves. A person who needs pink light may well need an essential oil with 'pink' vibrations. There is no essential oil that is literally pink in colour, but there are oils who vibration can appropriately be called 'pink'. ('The Healing Energy of Plants' will look at this in more detail.)

The therapist chooses a particular colour, sound, aroma, etc., because its vibration corresponds to something needed by the person seeking help. This may be in order to gently change an existing vibration, to add something that is lacking, or to strengthen what is already present, but the eventual aim is always to bring about a state of harmony for, as we have seen, dis-harmony can bring about disease.

Some practitioners working in the area of vibrational healing use tangible substances and hand-on techniques, others do not, but the one thing they all have in common is that they aim to alter vibrations or energy-patterns by one means or another. Among the therapies or systems sharing this subtle approach we find the Dr. Bach Flower Remedies, other Flower Essences and Gem Elixirs, homeopathy, acupuncture, crystal healing, Chakra balancing, radionics, spiritual healing and, of course, Subtle Aromatherapy.

Some of these make use of materials or instruments to mediate the healing energy in some way while some are concerned with 'pure' energy.

When an acupuncturist places needles in carefully chosen meridian points, the aim is not to affect the place where the needle is inserted, but to influence the flow of ch'i (energy) in the meridian. Meridians cannot be identified in the same way as a network of nerves or blood vessels. From a materialist point of view they do not exist, and yet this is a powerful system of healing. The vibrational state of the patient's ch'i is altered, and it is the ch'i which acts upon the physical body to bring about healing.

Even when the treatment involves ingesting a remedy, such as a homeopathic remedy or a flower essence, this is not given with the aim of directly acting on a particular organ or body system. In fact, scientifically-minded folk argue that neither of these treatments is capable of influencing the physical body because neither of them contain any measurable part of the flower, mineral or other substance from which they were prepared. All the same, physical healing takes place, if that is what is needed. Why? Because these remedies embody within them the healing vibrations of the plant or other originating material, and it is these vibrations which heal. They do not directly affect the physical matter that composes our bodies, but restore harmony in the subtle body, and once that is done, physical healing usually follows.

When we look at Subtle Aromatherapy, the situation is a little different, because essential oils are very concentrated plant extracts, capable of having a considerable and direct effect on the physical body (indeed, of doing great harm if misused). When they are used in the ways common to traditional aromatherapy they enter the bloodstream and have a demonstrable effect on the body (though nobody would deny the great psychological benefit of traditional aromatherapy). For this to become Subtle Aromatherapy, the oils need to be handled in a completely different way. The traditional aromatherapist works with very small amounts of essential oil, and dilutes them to around 3% for most applications, but to make the transition from physical aromatherapy to subtle energy work, these small amounts have to be reduced still further. An essential oil dilution of half to 1% is well below the concentration that most authorities consider necessary to have any physical effect.

In fact, the therapist may not apply any oil at all to the recipient's skin but work some distance off the body. Theoretically, this should have no effect at all. To understand why it does, it is necessary to consider the nature of essential oils.

These are very complex compounds, with many different substances made in the plant cells combining to produce the particular aroma and properties of the oil that is unique to that plant. These compounds are made up of aromatic molecules, each of which has its individual rate of vibration, and it is the vibration of these molecules that enable the olfactory cells in our noses detect smells. This is a physical vibration, comparable to those of light and sound. But essential oils also carry from their parent plants vibrations that convey something of the life-energy of the plant and it is this energy that we draw upon in Subtle Aromatherapy.

You might think of this as a higher form of vibration. Going back to the musical analogy I used earlier, you could say that these vibrations resonate at a much higher octave.

The colours, textures and aromas of essential oils may guide us in understanding their subtle properties but it is that other energy, that higher vibration which comes into play when we dilute the oils beyond the point where they are likely to have a physical effect. Although the dilutions are nowhere near as tiny as those used in homeopathy, a similar principle can be seen at work.

The other vital difference between traditional and Subtle Aromatherapy lies in the therapist's intent. By focusing upon the subtle action of the oils, we can bring them into play.

This brings us to the role of thought in vibrational healing. Thoughts themselves are a form of vibration. I am not thinking here of brain rhythms, or the activity of brain cells, which are actual physical phenomena but of the action of the mind which is intangible. Yet thought is one of the most powerful of all forms of energy.

'Thought precedes Form' is an awesome concept and a true one. Nothing that has ever been created by mankind, from the crudest flint axe-head to the noblest symphony, has been made without the maker first conceiving it in thought. Thought can kill and thought can heal.

Negative thoughts produce negative energy which manifests as discordant vibrations in the subtle body and this discord is quite capable of producing dis-ease. Conversely, positive thought produces harmonious energy.

If the human mind holds such potential, consider what is possible to that greater Mind which may be called God, the Buddha-mind, the Universal Consciousness. It is when we put aside our individual minds and allow that Mind to work through us that we truly become channels of healing.

CHAPTER 3

Subtle Anatomy

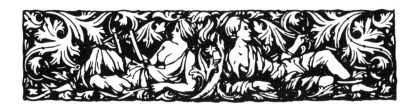

Every living thing – plant, animal and human – has a subtle anatomy which co-exists with its physical structure. It is this that makes Subtle Aromatherapy and all vibrational healing possible.

Throughout history mankind has found different ways of exploring, describing and working with this subtle anatomy. Probably the three best understood models, and those that are the most used in vibrational healing at the present day are the meridian system used in acupuncture, shiatsu and acupuncture, the theory of Chakra energy and the human aura, or energy field. Of these, the meridians have perhaps the least relevance to Subtle Aromatherapy although a small number of aromatherapists apply essential oil to specific meridian points in order to influence the ch'i (energy). The theory of Yin and Yang, which also forms part of Chinese medicine has been much more widely adopted by Western therapists.

The complete theory behind the practice of acupuncture and its related healing systems, is extremely complex and reflects the philosophy of Taoism. It embraces the ideas of the Five Elements, Earth, Metal, Water, Wood and Fire, of Yin and Yang, of ch'i as well as the meridians, which are the channels through which ch'i flows. All these factors are delicately inter-related.

Ch'i is the Chinese name for the life-force or subtle energy that permeates the Universe and sustains all living things. At birth, we bring a store of ch'i with us into physical existence, which is called our 'Before-Heaven Ch'i'. During our life, we may acquire more ch'i from our breath, food, specific exercises and spiritual practices and this is called 'After-Heaven Ch'i'. Ch'i is distributed throughout our bodies via the meridians, of which there are twelve.

Each meridian is connected with a particular organ or system of the body, although their relationship with the organs is as much symbolic as physical. Liver, for example, relates as much to anger as to the actual organ. Each organ also has one of the Five Elements associated with it, which expresses something about the energy-qualities of that organ. All are inter-connected, and the state of ch'i in one organ and its meridian will affect that in the next organ, as well as being influenced by it in turn.

The meridians function in pairs, with each pair being made up of one Yin and one Yang meridian. Ch'i moves from the head towards the feet through the Yang meridians on the back of the body, and from feet to head through the Yin meridians on the front.

The notion of Yin and Yang is one of the most widely understood (and maybe the most frequently mis-understood!) aspects of Chinese medicine and has been incorporated into many other subtle healing systems. In aromatherapy, it is possible to classify essential oils as Yin and Yang, though such classifications do not always stand up to close scrutiny. We can also assess the energy state of the people we work with as less or more Yin or Yang, and this is sometimes a useful indication of their current treatment needs.

The idea of Yin and Yang is a way of describing opposite and complementary states of energy, Yang being thought of as hot, dry active, outgoing and Yin as cold, damp, passive, introspective, etc., though these are relative rather than absolute states. There is some Yin in everything Yang and some Yang in all that is Yin, and the balance constantly changes.

Although, as I have said, Subtle Aromatherapy makes but little use of the Chinese model, some knowledge of the underlying principles can enrich our understanding of subtle energy. It is impossible to do justice to the whole philosophy here, and to those who would know more I recommend Ted Kaptchuk's classical work 'The Web That Has No Weaver'.

An equally ancient way of describing subtle energy is the Indian theory of Chakras, or energy centres in the body, and this has been embraced by many of the newer systems of vibrational healing. It has particular relevance to Subtle Aromatherapy, as many essential oils affect chakra energy, strengthening, decreasing or balancing as needed. Crystal healers, too, work with these energies, relating a variety of crystals or gemstones to each chakra and these two systems can be used together to wonderful affect by using crystals and essentials oils that have similar actions, each enhancing the activity of the other.

The word 'Chakra' is Sanskrit, meaning 'wheel' and it conveys not only the idea of a circle but also of turning, for the energy in the chakras is constantly revolving. There are many chakras situated throughout the body, many hundred in fact, though for the purposes of healing, visualization and meditation most people work with the seven major chakras situated on the midline of the body (Figure 1) while some include further chakras in the subtle bodies in the area above the crown of the head. These are the chakras with which I shall mainly be concerned in this book, although I shall also touch briefly on those in the hands, feet and knees, as these have some relevance in Subtle Aromatherapy.

Having just referred to the major chakras being situated on the midline of the body, I must clarify this before going any further: these chakras are often described in words as being located at various points along the spine, while in charts and pictures they are usually shown on the front of the body. In fact, each chakra should be thought of as extending right through the body from front to back at the level indicated. Not only that, but the energy of each chakra extends well beyond the visible body of matter into the subtle bodies or aura.

Each chakra has associated with it a particular element, colour, sound and shape that expresses something about the vibration of that centre. The colours, in particular, are often an indication of how essential oils relate to individual

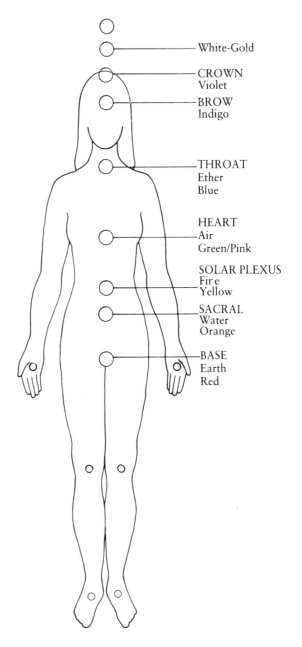

White-Gold

CROWN
Violet

BROW
Indigo

THROAT
Ether
Blue

HEART
Air
Green/Pink

SOLAR PLEXUS
Fir e
Yellow

SACRAL
Water
Orange

BASE
Earth
Red

Figure 1

chakras. Some people also attribute to each chakra an endocrine gland which that chakra is thought to influence. This is a relatively recent idea – I say 'relatively' because although it is not particularly new, it has been around for only a fraction of the 4,000 years or so that chakra energy has been understood! The endocrine gland theory has partly displaced the original system of associating each of the five lower chakras with one of the five elements: Earth, Water, Fire, Air and Ether, and I prefer to work within that framework as it has more relevance to Subtle Aromatherapy.

In this context, 'Ether' might better be called Space, The Heavens or The Formless, any of which comes a little nearer to the meaning of the original Sanskrit. In alchemical terms this substance is called 'quintessence' which has interesting connotations for the aromatherapist, as this word is sometimes used as an alternative (though somewhat 'unscientific') term for essential oils.

The distinctive vibration of each of the seven major chakras relates to a particular area of human experience, from our basic physical survival to our highest aspirations. Working with essential oils to heal and harmonize chakra energy can help individuals to achieve their highest potential. This is such a major area of Subtle Aromatherapy that I have devoted a chapter to it, and in that chapter you will find the major chakras described in greater detail. Even so, I have omitted much ancient knowledge, though only because it is not immediately relevant to our work with essential oils.

Much of what I have left out is to do with the symbolism of the Sanskrit alphabet, Hindu deities and Tantra, all of which were part of the ancient understanding of the chakras. The system has been modified in many ways over the millennia, as it was adopted into different cultures, and will undoubtedly continue to undergo subtle changes as Western healers and therapists bring their own outlook, philosophies and the needs of their 20th century clients to this ancient tradition. Despite this, an understanding of the origins of the system is enriching. There are many books about the chakras, and further reading is worthwhile if you choose to work in this area of Subtle Aromatherapy.

Both of these systems originate from a specific culture, but one that is equally ancient and apparently universal is the idea of the human aura. (Not only human, as animals certainly have an aura, and so do plants, as described elsewhere in this book.) Attempts to depict the aura are found in art as diverse as ancient Navajo rock paintings and Christian icons, as well as Persian, Japanese and Indian art, sometimes as a glow, or nimbus, surrounding the whole of a Deity or spiritual master, more often as the familiar halo surrounding the head.

The aura is sometimes described as an energy-field and sometimes as the subtle body, or more precisely as a series of subtle bodies. The several bodies, or layers of the aura have been described by different names at various times and by differing schools of thought which can become confusing. The names I use (Figure 2) are probably the most widely understood today, though they will not always correspond to those in earlier writings.

A minority of psychically-gifted people are able to see the auras of others, but virtually everybody working in subtle healing can sense the aura in non-visual ways. It is not difficult to feel with your hands the energy emanations, especially of the Etheric and Astral bodies. (If you have not yet experienced this, you may like to try the exercise described in the following chapter.) Such experiences confirm all the earlier descriptions of the human aura, as to shape, density, etc.

The overall form of the aura in a state of harmony and balance is egg-shaped, while within that ovoid the denser layers approximate more to the outline of the physical body. The size and shape fluctuate according to the mental,

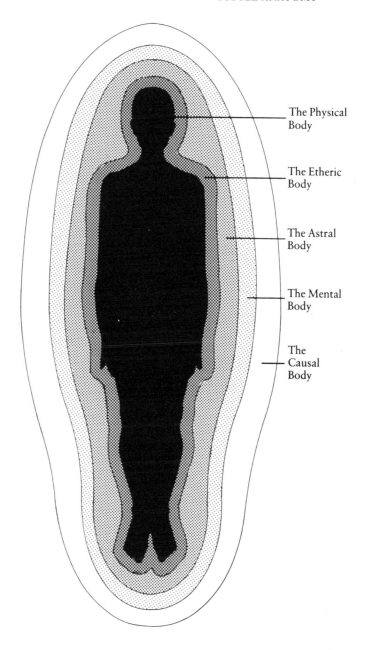

Figure 2

physical, emotional and spiritual health of the individual with the aura shrinking, becoming lop-sided, ragged or developing holes when energy is depleted or disturbed in any way.

There is less consensus regarding colours in the aura, there being many different descriptions of the colours and a variety of interpretations of what each colour may signify. What is universally agreed, though, is that the colours within the aura are clear and transparent but can become clouded or darkened by dis-ease and other factors.

Such changes in the state of the aura may relate to physical disease, shock, accidents, emotional trauma, drugs or thought-forms – both our own and others. Alcohol and smoking affect the aura, too, even one cigarette will darken it for an hour. Psychotropic drugs are often responsible for auric holes, which allow energy to leak out and leave the individual feeling very drained. You will see that I have referred to a number of physical factors that affect the state of the aura, but the converse is equally true. Changes in the subtle bodies influence the physical body, and can be felt by healers long before any sign of physical dis-ease is apparent.

It would be a mistake to think of the aura as something 'outside' or separate from the physical body, for the two are intricately connected. Auric energy permeates the physical body (and indeed, some believe that it is this which maintains life in the body).

The Causal body absorbs life-giving energy (ch'i or prana) which surrounds us at all times, and transmits it to the physical via the Mental, Astral and Etheric bodies, so giving both life and form to the physical, while the state of the physical body has a demonstrable effect on the subtle bodies.

This is most apparent in the Etheric body, which is the densest of the subtle bodies and the most closely integrated with the physical body. Changes in the physical state are immediately apparent as energy changes in the Etheric body, and therapists working with subtle energy are easily able to feel these changes and monitor them almost from one minute to the next during a healing session. The Astral body, though less dense, can also be sensed by many therapists and is often found to reflect very clearly the emotional state of the individual while some very sensitive people can sense all the subtle bodies, or layers of the aura and the corresponding changes which permeate right to its outer limits. Each band of the aura affects and is affected by the others, so that physical change or dis-ease will manifest first in the Etheric, then the Astral, the Mental and finally the Causal body. The 'memory' of an illness, accident or traumatic experience remains within the aura for some time, and will influence a person's well-being unless some form of healing, perhaps with essential oils and/or crystals is used to clear it completely.

Conversely, disease and other physical events are fore-shadowed in the outer layers of the aura before manifesting in the denser layers and the physical body, and healing the aura can prevent them ever becoming felt at a physical level. External influences make themselves felt first in the Causal body particularly when it is damaged or weakened in any way. We may imagine a kind of 'skin' protecting the whole aura from negative energies and it is when this is damaged that a variety of dark influences can infiltrate the aura, just as infection enters the physical body where the skin is broken. In particular, negative thought-forms 'infect' the outer layer of the aura, where a few very psychically-gifted people can actually see them in the form of pictures.

When the outer protective layer of the aura is breached, energy can flow out, as well as in and people who do have holes in their auras become very depleted in energy, and some of them – often quite unintentionally – try to make up for this by taking energy from others. Such people are sometimes referred to as 'psychic vampires' which can be a little unkind as such activity is almost always unconscious and beyond their control. All the same, we have all met people who leave us feeling drained, and this is the reason why. Everybody engaged in subtle healing work should be very aware of this, and use some form of self-protection before every healing session, as those in need of healing are frequently the very ones who are depleted in their auric energy.

One of the major benefits of auric massage and crystal healing is in maintaining the health of the 'skin' and repairing any damage to it as soon as possible. Bringing essential oils into the aura will always affect the energy-state, and by selecting the most appropriate oil we can energise or calm, clean, 'disinfect' and heal the aura. Auric massage, chakra work and combining crystal healing with essential oils are all valid methods of doing this while some healers simply channel healing energy via their hands.

Visualization, chanting, meditation and affirmations can also influence the state of the aura. We have seen how negative thought-forms can harm the aura and it is just as true to say that positive thought can heal it. Visualization, affirmations and some kinds of meditation are all ways of focusing positive thought. 'Thought precedes Form' is a profoundly true statement and we influence our health, both physical and subtle, by our thoughts. If we have mean, miserable, fearful, selfish or other unhelpful thoughts, they permeate the subtle bodies, and can eventually lead to physical ill-health. Conversely, positive thought promotes good health and can even reverse illness. We can improve our health, relationships, prosperity and virtually every aspect of our lives through thought.

Thought is one form of vibration, and thus changes the vibration in each of the subtle bodies for better or for worse.

Chanting is another form of vibration, perhaps a more obvious one as it is possible to physically feel the resonance of the sounds. This, too, can have a very beneficial and invigorating influence on the subtle bodies. Chanting, meditation, prayer and all forms of spiritual exercise strengthen the aura and the auras of spiritually advanced beings are enormous. That of the Buddha was said to be 200 miles in extent.

Various attempts have been made to explain the phenomenon of the aura in scientific terms, the most popular of which is the notion of electro-magnetic energy. While it is certainly true that such energy does surround every body, and can be detected and even demonstrated by such means as Kirlian photography and the more recently developed technique known as AuraVision, it is unlikely that this is the only kind of energy involved. The Etheric body may be composed partly of electro-magnetic energy, since it has the most immediate interaction with the physical.

The aura is sometimes described as being formed of ch'i, or prana, both terms for the life-force that surrounds and pervades all living things. I find this description satisfying, for it sums up the whole relationship between the physical body, the subtle bodies and the universe in which they co-exist.

CHAPTER 4

The Role of the Healer

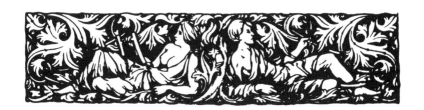

It may help in defining the role of the healer or therapist in vibrational medicine if we first look at what is implied by the word 'healing'.

Healing is power that channels through one person to another.

Healing can mean many things:

- Moving towards being whole.
- Helping people to shift blocks that stop them moving forwards.
- Opening up potentials.
- Restoring physical health.
- Bringing different aspects of the personality together.
- Helping people to be in tune with the rest of Creation – to be at one with the Planet.

Whichever of these aspects of healing we consider – and they are but a few of the possibilities – the role of the healer is to focus and direct the most appropriate healing vibrations towards the person seeking healing. As an analogy, think of a lens which focuses light on a single point. The lens is not light, but the light must pass through the lens to the point where it is needed. Without light, the lens has no function. Healing energy surrounds us at all times, but most often needs to be focused in some way towards people who need help. So we can think of the healer as the lens which focuses healing energy where it is needed.

How he or she does so will depend on the system of healing involved. This focusing may involve conscious, intellectual decisions based on formal training or it may be purely intuitive, though the two are by no means mutually exclusive. Richard Wagner wrote 'Intuitive decisions are good, but you make them after equipping yourself with all the information possible in the area in which the decisions are to be made'. He was talking about composing, but his remarks are just as applicable to many areas of vibrational medicine.

37

For example, the homeopath or the acupuncturist has studied for several years in order to amass the necessary information about the repertoire of remedies or the network of meridian points, and, theoretically at least, could base all treatment decisions on this fund of intellectual knowledge. But if you ask any practitioner, he or she will say that a measure of intuition enters into such decisions as well. Similarly, the aromatherapist must know all the properties of a wide repertoire of essential oils, their uses, the situations in which any oil should not be used, and so forth but the final choice of oil will involve the therapist's intuitive response to the client's needs at that moment. This is equally true whether we are thinking of traditional or Subtle Aromatherapy, even though there will probably be greater reliance on intuition in the latter. The secret, I think, lies in gaining so thorough an intellectual grasp of the techniques and materials of one's chosen therapy that they become second nature. At that point, intuition can come into play.

At the other end of the scale, the spiritual healer uses no 'tools' or method to bring about healing, but is simply willing to be an open channel through which healing energy can flow.

Whether an individual chooses to work with essential oils, with crystals, flower essences, homeopathic remedies, acupuncture needles or any of the other possibilities that fall within the broad description of 'vibrational healing' will depend very much on the personality, background, hopes and dreams of that person. The highly intuitive person may opt for crystals or one or other of the plant-based therapies, while the more intellectually inclined might choose the demanding study needed to master acupuncture or homeopathy. Some people discover their healing ability at an early stage and are quite happy to work with nothing more than their hands, while others feel more confident if they have tangible 'tools' and an identifiable system within which to operate.

We can rejoice in the fact that there are so many options in vibrational healing because, just as different therapists will be drawn to different ways of working, so will the people who need healing. Somebody who is sceptical about 'healing' might be perfectly happy to book an aromatherapy session, because the oils and the hand-on massage are something solid that they can trust, while another who thinks crystals are just a bit too strange to be involved with, would be quite happy receiving acupuncture.

One great healer who I feel very privileged to have met, told me that she works with colour, sound, aromatherapy and the Dr. Bach Flower Remedies because they offer something for each of the five senses and different people respond better to one or the other.

But even when essential oils, crystals, needles, remedies or any other aid to healing are used, the person and personality of the healer or therapist is still a major factor and if we think of the healer as a lens or channel, it is obvious that nothing can pass through if the lens is clouded or the channel silted up. So therapists who wish to work at a subtle level must be prepared to work on themselves to ensure that the lens is clear and bright, and that energy can flow freely through the channel.

All manner of influences can impede the free flow of healing energy: illness, emotional trauma, wrong motivation, lack of belief in one's own ability to channel healing. Even poor posture or lack of exercise can sometimes be a block. Everybody who works in the area of vibrational healing will know that they sometimes have days, or longer periods of time, when they feel depleted, blocked or unable to offer healing for one reason or another. I think it is important to recognise such times, and get whatever help is needed rather than trying to struggle on. Get somebody else to give you some healing, a massage, a crystal healing, or a big hug. Better still, make sure you allow yourself to be nurtured as often as you need, without waiting until you feel drained.

Sometimes, energy blocks arise from very old traumas, even from past-life experiences, and then it is important that the healer, or embryo healer, gets good professional help and guidance.

Some form of psychotherapy might be needed to shift old pains, or regression if past-life experiences seem to be implicated. Take great care when choosing a therapist to find one who is sympathetic with your ultimate aim of healing. Certain schools of psychotherapy reduce everything to a mental/material level and would regard a wish to heal as a problem in itself!

Most of the work that is needed, though, has to be done by the individual. To become a clear channel through which healing energy can pass may entail a regular meditation practice, or it might mean 'cleaning up your act' on a physical level by giving up smoking, cutting down on alcohol or taking more exercise. Harmonious forms of exercise such as yoga and swimming and some kinds of dancing are very beneficial. Chanting is another tool for shifting energy and clearing away old blocks. The cosmic sound AUM (OM) embraces the beginning and the end of everything, and is a particularly powerful instrument of change. You might like to try chanting the OM for a period of time each day. Early morning is probably the best time, and keep it up for as long as you can manage. Twenty minutes is probably the least time that has an effect at a deep level, and if you can manage to chant for longer, that is even better.

Yes, we've all met chain-smoking, coffee-swigging healers but it's not a good idea to take one of them as your role-model! Perhaps they exist to remind us that healing is a mystery which nobody completely understands.

If you are completely new to the field of Subtle Aromatherapy, you might find it helpful to have some exercises for learning to recognise and work with vibrational energy. Perhaps you are a traditional aromatherapist who wants to work more in the vibrational area, or maybe you practise some other physical therapy and wish to incorporate some aspects of Subtle Aromatherapy into your present work. Or you may not be a practising therapist at all, but yet feel drawn towards the healing arts.

These three simple exercises are what I give to my own students at the very beginning of their training. You'll need a partner if you want to try them out.

For the first exercise sit facing your partner (Figure 3). Cross-legged on the floor is best, but if you really can't manage it, two chairs facing would do. You must be near enough to touch each other's hands without leaning forward.

Put your left hand on your knee, palm facing upwards and ask your partner to do the same. Now place your right hand, palm facing downwards, over your partner's hand and ask your partner to do this, too. Close your eyes and take some deep, slow breaths. As you breathe in, imagine that healing energy is pouring into you with the breath, and as you breathe out imagine yourself sending energy out through the palm of your right hand to your partner, at the same time receiving energy from your partner through the palm of your left hand. Continue doing this until you both feel that there is a continuous circuit of energy flowing between you. Now, very slowly, you should both lift your right hand, and see how high you can take it without losing the connection between you. Move your hand slowly up and down to see if you can find the point at which the connection is strongest. Gradually bring your hands back into contact again, and break the circuit by moving your right hands out sharply to the side.

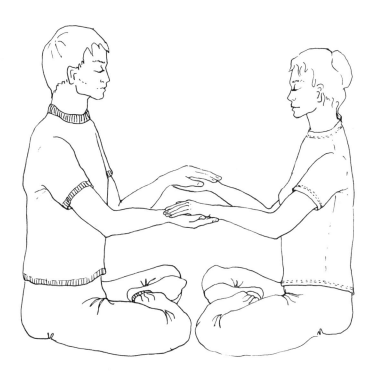

Figure 3

You will probably want to spend a few minutes discussing with your partner whatever sensations you felt. Some people experience warmth, or a tingling sensation in their hands. This may be stronger in one hand than the other, and it may be felt very strongly in the centre of the palm or in the fingertips. Others feel a pull rather like that of a pair of magnets, and occasionally there may be a cool sensation, rather than warmth. All of these are manifestations of energy passing between your hands, and it is this energy that heals.

For the next exercise you and your partner need to sit back to back (Figure 4). Sit up as straight as you can so that as much of your spine as possible is in contact with your partner's spine. Spend a few moments breathing slowly and then focus your attention on your partner's back. See how much you can find out about your partner through his or her back, try to sense whether there are any areas that are tense, tired or painful (not necessarily in the back) and if you find any, mentally direct healing energy to that place. At the same time, feel open to receiving healing energy from your partner into any needy areas of your own body.

Five minutes is long enough for this exercise, and once again you will want to give each other some feedback. See whether you were right about the areas of each other's bodies that you thought needing some healing, and whether any healing took place.

The third exercise is one I call the 'energy trace'. For this you will need your partner to lie face down. (If you are already a practitioner and have a treatment couch available, it is much easier to have your partner lie on the couch.) Put your left hand at the top of your partner's neck, so that the little-finger side just touches the base of your partner's skull. Now hold your right hand at the bottom of your partner's back over the base of the spine and about an inch above the body. Allow your right hand to move slowly towards the

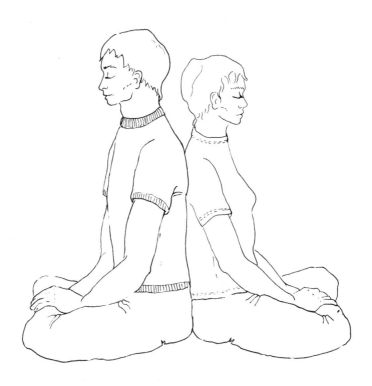

Figure 4

top of your partner's spine, until it meets your left hand. Try to feel that your hand is being pulled, rather than that you are moving it yourself. As you do this, be aware of your partner's energy. Note any change in what your moving hand can feel, any areas where your hand moves faster or slower, any sensations of cold or warmth and anything else you pick up. It may be helpful to close your eyes.

If you feel that any area of your partner's back is giving you 'distress signals', that energy is blocked at some point along the spine, or is lacking anywhere, spend a little time making stroking movements, or any other movement you feel intuitively to be needed, over that area. Then do the energy trace again and note whether there is any change. For example, if you found a place where your hand moved very slowly, energy may well be blocked at that point. Stroking movements towards the head will often move the block, and when you repeat the energy trace you'll find that your hand no longer slows down at that point.

You can do an energy trace with a clothed partner, but if you find it difficult, try it with your partner's back un-covered and a little massage oil. In this case let your hand glide very lightly on the surface of the skin – but only just touch. You can incorporate an energy trace at the end of a massage session or an auric massage, as well as using it as a training exercise. You might also try it again later after reading the chapter on Chakra Energy, and see if you can identify the chakras as you move your hand up the spine.

Everybody engaging in vibrational healing needs some form of protection to avoid picking up negative energies from clients. You may already have a favourite way of protecting yourself, but if not here are some suggestions.

The simple visualization for closing the chakras, which you will find in that chapter, is a good protection, and takes only a few seconds to accomplish once you are familiar with it. Other people have other ways they like to close their chakras, and if you know one already, stick with your own favourite. Some people wrap themselves in an invisible but protective cloak, while others like to surround themselves with a purple flame. I know of one healer who mentally zips himself into a garment he calls his 'cosmic babygro'! It may sound daft, but it works for him, and that is all that matters. My own favourite is the white light meditation, which I share with you now.

Sit in any comfortable position and see in your mind's eye a brilliant white light shining in the sky above you. Rays of white light beam down to a point in the centre of your forehead, and pour into your body. Imagine that your body is like an empty vase, and the white light is filling it up. Feel the sensation of this light filling every part of your body. When you feel that you are entirely filled with white light, imagine that the beam of light now becomes soft and flexible, so that you can wrap it around yourself like a scarf. Begin to wrap this light around you until you are entirely enclosed in it like a cocoon. Remember that, because it is a scarf of light, it will not restrict you in any way, and that when you are ready to move you can do so freely. Once you feel you are surrounded by the light, you can let the beam go back to its source. Think of this source of light as representing whatever is most sacred to you, and give thanks for its protection.

Now that you are completely filled and surrounded by white light, no negative energy can harm you. You can take the white light with you, whatever you are doing and for as long as you feel you need its protection.

This meditation takes far less time to carry out than it does to describe, and if it appeals to you, you will find that you can do it simply and quickly before each healing session.

It is also good to ground yourself before giving healing – in fact this is true even if you are simply giving physical aromatherapy. Make sure that your stance is firm, with your feet apart, your knees relaxed and your back straight. Be aware of your centre of gravity at the hara (the lower abdomen). Imagine roots from the soles of your feet extending down into the Earth and send two or three breaths out through your feet into your roots. Remember, even if you are working indoors on an upper floor, that the building itself has foundations going firmly into the ground and that you can ground and connect to Earth through them.

You will also need to think about cleansing at the end of every healing session. Just as the physical therapist washes his or her hands between each client, we need to shed any vibrational influence from one person before we engage in energy work with another. Hold your hands under cold, running water and let it pour over your wrists, as you do so visualizing all negativity pouring away with the water. Do this after every session. If you want to wash your hands in warm, soapy water, do this after the cold.

If you give several healing sessions following each other, it is good at the end of the day to visualize yourself being cleansed by a shower of water, too. You could imagine a shower of golden rain pouring over you, gently washing away all negativity, all fatigue or you might prefer to imagine wading into a stream and standing beneath a waterfall: feel the water cascading down over your head and shoulders, streaming down your body taking with it all your weariness and negativity, which is then swept away down the river to join the great ocean where it is transmuted.

You will notice that each of these cleansing techniques involves running water, whether in reality or in visualization. This is because water is cleansing psychically as well as physically. Cold water moves energy, but hot water fixes it.

Finally, I want to encourage you to use your healing ability. Many people have a great potential for healing and are afraid to use it.

In fact, I believe that every person on Earth is able to heal, if only they allowed themselves to do so. An altruistic motivation, a genuine desire to be of service, is the most important factor.

If you truly want to heal you will find that you can.

CHAPTER 5

The Healing Energies of Plants

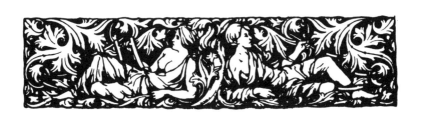

Human beings have drawn upon the healing power of plants since time immemorial, as well as using them for food, clothing, shelter, pigments and personal adornment. Indeed, plants almost certainly provided some of the earliest aesthetic experiences for mankind as consciousness evolved into something we may call human. As well as the visual delight of a beautiful flower, we can imagine how much those far-distant men and women savoured the perfume of aromatic plants, for their olfactory sense was much sharper than ours.

It is hardly surprising, then, that plants are central to both the medical and spiritual practices of mankind as far back as we have any evidence. Indeed, in many traditions there is no distinction between medicine and religion: the shaman is both priest and doctor. The American Indian concept of 'medicine' is an example: medicine, to the Native American is not limited to the cure of physical ills, but embraces the spiritual life as well as serving to connect the user to the Earth and to all other living creatures.

In most modern societies medicine and religion have become separated, but the use of plants persists in many religions as incense and sometimes anointing oils and of course plants play an important role in medicine, both orthodox and alternative. The ability of plants to heal physical dis-ease is acknowledged and thoroughly researched: in many instances we know exactly which molecules within a plant serve to bring about the healing process (and many synthetic drugs are 'carbon copies' of these plant molecules, though they lack the life-force or healing energy of the real plant).

In subtle aromatherapy, though, as in other forms of vibrational healing such as homeopathy and the flower remedies, we draw on less tangible properties of plants to help in healing and transformation. In doing so we come closer to the shaman's sacred smoke, or the priest using incense than to the doctor, herbalist or traditional aromatherapist.

When plants, or extracts from them, are used in vibrational healing it is the vibration or subtle energy of the plant which is the healing factor and this is harder to explain or examine than the physical properties of medicinal plants. Each plant has its own particular vibration, something unique to offer us for our wholeness. So how can we set about discovering these subtle healing properties?

We can take a look at how plants have been used in the past, in shamanistic traditions, in the ceremonial of many different religions, their symbolism in art, their meaning in myth and folklore. We can develop our own intuition and learn from the intuitive knowledge of others and we can draw on the large body of information that has been revealed in recent decades by direct channelling. Finally, we can study the plants themselves, for they can tell us much about their hidden abilities.

Studying earlier uses of plants does not mean merely following precedent. When human beings call upon plants for their healing power, some kind of interaction between plant and man takes place. Marcel Lavabre suggests that plants have a 'memory' of the ways in which human beings have used them in the past and that each time we use them for the same purpose this reinforces the plants' memory of that purpose. He expresses this idea by applying the theory of the morphogenetic field to healing plants. He likens a morphogenetic field to a landscape with hills and valleys, rivers and streams where each river and valley represents a flow of information. When some totally new information is added it makes a tiny furrow on the landscape, but every time this new information is used, the furrow gets deeper until eventually it becomes a deep valley. Every person who uses this information makes it easier for the next person to learn it. For example, when computers were first invented it took people a long time to learn how to use them: now there are computers in the classrooms at infant schools. So, each time we work with plant vibrations for healing, we make it easier for that plant to be used for healing by others.

Learning how the healing energies of plants helped people in the past is a valid starting point for our work today. Another, which also links us to ancient usage, is the healing and mystical practices of peoples who have preserved a shamanistic tradition: such as the Native Americans, Maoris and Australian aborigines. For example, the Native Americans have preserved the ancient practice of burning aromatic plants to produce a scented smoke, which they call 'smudging' and this is nothing other than a form of Subtle Aromatherapy.

References to plants, especially 'magical' plants in myths, fairytales and folklore can throw up valuable clues as can the symbolism of plants in art, poetry and the writings of mystics. References to flowers and plants and the beliefs associated with them can be found everywhere, and anything that you can learn about a plant will enrich your understanding of it and hence of how it can heal. Astrology also offers some insights: Culpeper and other herbalists assigned a ruling planet to each plant and those planets are named after the gods of classical antiquity – Mars, Venus, Mercury and so on. Studying the personality or attributes of these gods will tell you something about the plants under their rule. Read gardening books and those that describe the flora of various regions, especially if they are well illustrated.

At first, you will take in this information at an intellectual level, but try to absorb it, to make it part of you, so that you can draw on it intuitively whenever you use an essential oil.

The best way to learn about plant energies, though, is to study the plants themselves. Try to spend time near plants and be sensitive to them. Dr. Edward Bach found each of the 38 plants that make the Flower Remedies which he pioneered by tuning intuitively to the plant to discover what it could offer to mankind. People in Alaska, Australia, California, Scotland and elsewhere are currently developing new Flower Remedies in just the same way, although in some instances the information about which plants to use and where to look for them is being directly channelled.

The shape, texture, colour, habit of growth, preferred climate or altitude and, of course, the smell of a plant can all tell you something about its healing energies, both on the physical and subtle planes.

For example, colour may suggest an affinity with a particular healing Ray or with a certain Chakra. This may be the colour of the flower, leaves, fruit or of the essential oil itself. Although only a minority of essential oils are coloured, the colours of those that are, are always a significant factor in understanding their subtle energies. Dark colours, such as browns and deep reds (as in Patchouli or Myrrh, for example) often denote a slow vibration, grounding energy and an affinity with the Base Chakra while the Green of Bergamot and Inula or the blue of certain Camomile oils indicate a higher vibratory rate and a connection with the Heart and Throat Chakras respectively.

If you are familiar with the theory of Top, Middle and Base notes which is used both in perfumery and traditional aromatherapy to describe essential oils by comparing them to notes on the musical stave, you can use this as an indication of what to expect from a particular oil in terms of vibrations.

A plant that hugs the ground will have a very different energy from one that constantly pushes up towards the sky, and the vibrations of spiky, thorny or rough-textured plants will differ from those that are soft and rounded. Take Lavender and Rosemary for example: they are very closely related botanically but differ considerably in their healing properties. Spiky Rosemary yields a lively, energising oil, while the gently rounded cushion of the Lavender bush expresses just as eloquently the calming and balancing powers of Lavender oil.

The oils we use most often to facilitate meditation mainly come from trees with aromatic woods or resins (and the resins and woods were used as incense long before oil distillation was invented). Consider trees in relation to the rest of the plant kingdom: their branches reach nearer to Heaven than any other plant, and their roots go deeper into the Earth. Thus the tree maintains perfect equilibrium. Nothing could be a more apt symbol of what we aim for in meditation.

Climate and altitude also influence plant vibrations and if you succeed in establishing a plant where conditions are different from its native habitat, both the vibration and the essential oil will change. For example, alpine or high-altitude Lavender has a much more refined and etherial energy than Lavender grown at lower altitudes, even though they are botanically identical plants.

The part of a plant from which the essential oil or other remedy is extracted is another important factor in under-standing its energy potential. Oils distilled from the root are often very grounding in nature, though there are some notable exceptions to this rule, such as Angelica.

Oils from the leaves and twigs range widely in their energy. Many relate to physical wellbeing, others act on the mental sphere, yet others are psychic protectors or cleansers. This relates to the enormous variety of sizes, shapes, colours and textures found among leaves: think of the soft, furry leaves of Sage and the finely divided, feathery foliage of Camomile for example.

Flowers represent the highest attainment of the plant kingdom and are often seen in art and poetry as symbols of perfection or of spiritual qualities: a Madonna Lily, a perfect Rose, a humble Violet, etc., so it is not surprising that the exquisite oils they yield have extremely refined vibrations with an affinity for the higher Chakras. Flowers themselves, ephemeral as they are, teach us many lessons about impermanence and non-attachment, they show us our true potential and invoke our highest spiritual response.

A number of oils are obtained from seeds and fruits, notably those of the Citrus family. These oils tend to be nurturing, feeding us on subtle levels just as fruits feed the physical body. They have a simple, cheerful quality to their energies and are often used as antidepressants in traditional aromatherapy.

Ideally, the best way to know plants is to grow them, which allows you to know the plant intimately, but of course this is not possible for everybody, nor with every plant, for some of our aromatics have special requirements as to soil and climate that even the keenest gardeners cannot reproduce. Even so, it helps to grow as many aromatic plants as you can. Many of them will do well in English gardens: Roses, Lavender, all the culinary herbs, Camomiles, some Jasmines and so forth. Jasmine does well as a houseplant, and any of the culinary herbs will grow in a window box. If you are fortunate enough to have a conservatory, you might even grow some of the citruses for their blossom. Whether or not you have a garden of your own, it is always a delight as well as a valuable learning time if you visit specialist herb gardens where you can see, smell and sometimes touch a wide range of aromatic plants.

These correlations between essentials oils and the different characteristics of the plants that produce them may seem somewhat simplistic, but they embody real truths. They are not entirely inflexible – you will always find some plants and oils that do not conform to the general pattern, but such is the complexity of Nature.

Another way of understanding plant energies is to become

aware of their auras. Every plant has an aura, just as we do. The vibration of a plant aura is extremely refined and indicates clearly the particular area of healing to which that plant is best fitted. It is quite easy to learn to feel them. It is probably best to start with a big, sturdy plant as its aura will be correspondingly robust and easy to detect. (The first plant aura I ever felt was that of a large rubber-plant and it was quite as big as that of some human friends. It was growing in a meditation centre, so maybe its aura was more developed than most!) Just hold your hands near the plant and move them gently away and nearer again, exactly as you would to tune in to the energy of another person.

Tree auras can be huge. In woodland they overlap each other which is why a walk in the woods can be a healing in itself. Find a tree that is not growing too close to any others and walk slowly towards it with your arms outstretched until you become aware of its energy. Another way to experience the energy of a tree is to sit with your back resting against its trunk and just allow yourself to be sensitive to what you can feel.

Every plant has its own Deva, or spirit guardian. Devas are of the same order of being as Angels and we might think of them as the guardian angels of the plants. The Devas play an important part in healing, acting as an intermediary between plants and humans, so think of them as friends and ask for their help whenever you need it and always thank the Deva as well as the plant afterwards. They gently influence the energy and vibrations of the plants. Most often, this was done long ago, when the plant was first evolving, but can happen at any time when there is a need for change. The most notable example of this in recent times is the giant vegetables that grew in the Findhorn gardens in the early days of the community there. As both the Earth's energies and mankind's needs in terms of subtle healing from plants are changing rapidly at the present time, we can expect to see rapid evolution in some plant species.

Children are very receptive to Devic energy and some very sensitive children may see them, though they are likely to refer to them as 'fairies'. To contact the Devas ourselves it helps if we put aside all preconceptions and approach plants with the open simplicity of children.

CHAPTER 6

Some Ways of Using Essential Oils at a Subtle Level

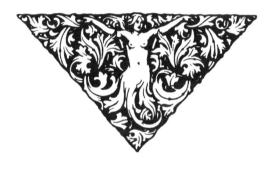

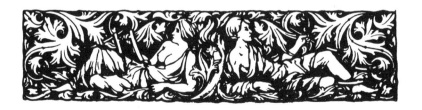

You can use essential oils for their subtle effects in any way you like! You need not be tied to any conventional method of application. You can use your imagination, be creative. After all, each of the accepted and tried ways of using essential oil was new once. What matters is your INTENT. Each time you use an essential oil for subtle or spiritual purposes, begin with a clear idea of what you aim to achieve and how you want the oil to help you. Invoke the help of the plant and its guardian spirit (Deva) and let the plant know why you need its help. (And don't forget to thank the plant afterwards.) Provided you do this with sincerity and humility, the method you use is secondary.

All the same, some methods have a long history of use for particular purposes and you may find them most helpful, at least initially. The longer you practise subtle aromatherapy, the more you attune yourself to the subtle energy of plants, the more likely you will be to discover or invent your own methods. The following are some ideas to help you as you start out on this path.

First, though, there are some fundamentals that apply whatever methods you may use.

1. Work Safely

In other words, be sure that you know and observe all the same safety rules that apply to the physical uses of essential oils. If you are already familiar with traditional aromatherapy you will know that, while the majority of oils can very safely be used by most people, there are a few oils which are genuinely dangerous, some that need to be used with caution, and certain groups of vulnerable people for whom essential oils must be chosen and used with special care. These include pregnant women, babies and children, people with epilepsy, those with high blood pressure, anybody who has received chemotherapy and anybody receiving ongoing treatment from a doctor or other qualified practitioner (such as a homeopath, medical herbalist or acupuncturist) for any illness or physical condition.

If you are not already thoroughly familiar with the physical properties of essentials oils, make sure that you learn something about them before you attempt to use the oils for subtle purposes. The fact that you are not looking to the oils for their physical effects will not make these effects inoperative: in other words, if I put a skin-irritant oil in a bath that I intend to use for ritual cleansing, it will sting my skin just as surely as if I merely wanted to wash.

Far more seriously, ignorance of the physical properties of essential oils could precipitate an epileptic fit in a susceptible person or cause a pregnant woman to lose her baby. It is also important to know such basic facts as whether a particular oil is sedative or stimulating. For example, Rosemary oil is a psychic protector; it is also a strong stimulant so if you use it during the evening you are likely to have a very disturbed night.

It is neither possible nor appropriate to go fully into all the physical properties of essential oils in this book. This information is available elsewhere, and I beg you not to overlook it in your eagerness to explore the more intuitive levels. I would refer you to my earlier book, 'Aromatherapy, an A-Z'. for guidance on properties and safety.

2. Use Very Little Oil

When you use essential oils for their subtle properties you will need far less than when you are looking for a physical effect. As a general rule, the smaller the amount of oil used, the more potent is its subtle effect. If you use the amounts and proportions of essential oil recommended for physical treatments, you will usually experience only a physical effect.

For example, in preparing an aromatic bath to ease tight muscles, you would use 6 to 8 drops of essential oil. To prepare a bath for ritual cleansing, you should use 3 drops or less.

If you decide to give a physical massage with the intent of evoking a subtle response, you should use only a 1% dilution of essential oil, rather than the usual 3%.

For other uses, I will mention the amount of oil needed as the book progresses. Please do not be tempted to use more than is indicated. It is very easy to 'swamp' the subtle effect by using more oil than is necessary.

3. Use Very Good Oils

Use the very best essential oils you can find. They will cost more than poorer quality oils initially, but you are only going to use minute amounts. Essential oils last for a very long time provided they are properly handled and stored, so you should think of each bottle as a treasured investment. Middling-quality oils may give satisfactory results in physical treatments (though even then I would not advise using them) but not in more subtle ways. They may have been distilled too quickly, or at too high a temperature with the result that some constituents will have been lost or destroyed. This inevitably alters the subtle vibration of the oil. Worse, there are some very poor quality oils offered for sale, and these sometimes include adulterations or outright synthetics which have nothing to do with aromatherapy of any kind at all.

If possible, use oils from plants that have been grown without chemicals (organically produced or wild plants) and extracted from the plant by distillation, expression or enfleurage rather than solvent extraction. In this way you can be sure that no chemical contaminants are present in the materials you use, either from the growing or the extraction methods. It goes without saying that any extraneous chemicals will affect the subtle energy of a plant.

There is more to organic growing, though, than simply avoiding chemical residues: plants grown this way are almost always healthier, more vigorous, more full of life energy than their chemically grown counterparts and this vigour is apparent in the oils distilled from them. You may perceive it in the strength and fullness of their aromas, but at the same time in a gentleness and in many delicate nuances of aroma that are not always apparent in other oils. The healing power of an oil relates directly to this vigour as well as to the oil's purity.

Suppliers of organic oils will be able to tell you which part of the plant is used (this can be very important), the method of extraction, the country of origin and sometimes the altitude or region where that makes a difference to the oil. They will also identify the plant by its botanical (Latin) name, which is the only way to be sure you are buying the exact oil you want for a specific purpose. Common names of plants, local nicknames and errors of translation can cause confusion but botanical names are understood all over the world.

Equally important is the fact that such oils will usually have been produced by people who treat the soil, the plants and the oils they yield with care and respect, even with love. We cannot expect to give or receive healing at the highest levels if our materials have been obtained by exploiting and poisoning our good Mother Earth.

4. Work Ethically

This area is perhaps harder to define than the first three but is, of course, the most important.

Conventional aromatherapy training emphasises, quite rightly, the great responsibility that the therapist bears when carrying out treatments that affect another person's body.

How much greater must be the responsibility when we work in ways that can affect our own and others' psyches? So I beg you to consider the following ideas very seriously before you embark on any work of this nature.

Do not try subtle aromatherapy techniques out of curiosity or 'for kicks'. Please embark on this work only if you, and any other person involved, has a genuine desire for healing, insight, personal or spiritual growth.

Do not try to use subtle aromatherapy to influence any other person without their knowledge or consent, with the exception of absent healing techniques. Even here, it is better if the person in need of healing knows that you are offering help in this way.

Never make any claim to heal physical illness through subtle aromatherapy. Physical healing MAY take place as a result, and in fact often does, but you should never envisage this as your sole or principal aim. True healing may sometimes lie in enabling a suffering person to approach death peacefully, even joyfully.

Never offer aromatherapy (traditional or subtle) to anybody who is seriously ill unless their doctor knows about it and has no objection.

Do not be tempted to use mood-altering oils to duck out of tough moments in your life. Remember that crisis can mean opportunity. Use the oils to support you at such times so that you can grow through and beyond crises. Similarly, if you use essential oils to facilitate personal or spiritual growth, do not expect them to replace inner effort. Growth can be hard work! The oils can help you in such work, but they can never replace it. They are not magic spells or a road to instant enlightenment.

Finally, always work from your Higher Self. It is so easy to let our little human personalities get in the way but all healing or subtle work needs to be undertaken with a pure and altruistic motivation. Dedicate your work to whatever represents the highest ideal in your personal belief system. You may call this ideal Christ, Buddha, God, the Highest Good or by whatever name is meaningful to you but it should always guide and illuminate your healing work.

Turning now to actual methods of working, let's begin by looking at how you can use the basic methods of conventional aromatherapy – massage, baths and burners – for subtle effect.

MASSAGE

Massage is fundamental to the practice of conventional aromatherapy and it can be a good starting point for the subtle aromatherapist. You might wish to start by simply bringing a subtle intent to your physical massage work. Invoke the higher levels of plant energy when you are choosing and preparing your oils, and be aware that the massage will then work for the receiver on levels beyond the mental and physical. Form a clear mental picture of the plant or plants whose oil you are about to use, and try to carry that picture in your mind while you are working. Ground and centre your own energies before you begin work. (If you don't know how to do this you can find some suggestions in another chapter.)

If the person you are going to massage is receptive to the idea of massage as subtle therapy, you can take the whole session on to a more refined energy level. Start by discussing with your friend what he or she is hoping to gain from this massage. This will guide you in your choice of oils, though if the two of you are well attuned to each other you will probably already have some intuitive feelings about the right oil to use. Tell your friend which oil or oils you have decided on, so that he or she is aware of the plant energy that is going to be present in the massage. Then both of you can form a mental picture of the plant and invoke its help. Some people like to meditate together for a short time before a massage session. If you do, you might choose to meditate on the plants and their healing powers.

Before you begin the massage, mix your chosen oil or oils in your carrier oil as usual, but using a much lower dilution than for a simple physical massage. One percent of essential oil, or even as little as a half percent is all you need. When you start the massage, omit any deep strokes, particularly if they are likely to feel uncomfortable to the receiver. Concentrate on light effleurage and long sweeping strokes, particularly those that influence energy flow (for example, strokes that follow a meridian). Let your hands come to rest on any area of the body that feels as if it needs special healing, and be aware of the healing energy flowing through your hands into your friend. Pay special attention to the extremities: hands, feet and head, drawing off any negative energy that may be present (and don't forget to give your hands a brisk shake each time you do so). At the end of the massage, include some strokes that do not touch the surface of the body (auric massage). Before beginning this phase of the massage, hold your hands above your friend's body and move them slowly, sensing any areas that feel cold, hot, blocked or troubled in any way, and make gentle stroking movements above any areas where you feel there is a need.

Don't worry if you have never done anything like this before – you'll be surprised how simply you can pick up such sensations. You might find it easier if you shut your eyes. If you really can't feel anything, try moving your hands nearer to or further away from your friend's body.

Always finish with some long, sweeping strokes from below the feet to above the head, at a little distance from the body. End by holding your friend's feet for a minute or more, to ground his or her energy and allow a gentle return to everyday reality. Allow plenty of time for your friend to rest and savour the experience and, if it feels appropriate, to discuss it with you. Don't forget to ground yourself at the end, too.

Massage offers several benefits in the field of subtle aromatherapy. Firstly, it serves as a valuable introduction to this area of work. It is the most familiar form of aroma-therapy, and both the therapist and the receiver may find it reassuring to work within this familiar framework initially. Secondly, people who are becoming more aware of subtle energy levels can sometimes get quite out of touch with their bodies (and may even see it as a virtue to do so!). The gentle physical context of massage helps us to stay grounded and human which, after all, is the only way we can function effectively on this planet. Thirdly, massage releases both physical tensions and emotional blocks, either of which can be a hindrance to growth: it is very difficult to meditate, visualize or soar to higher planes when your body is reminding you all-too-painfully of its presence! Remember that hatha yoga originated as a series of exercises to make the yogi better fitted physically to sit in meditation, sometimes for long periods.

RITUAL BATHS

Next to massage, bathing is the second most familiar way of using essential oils for their physical benefits and this method, too, can be adapted very simply to subtle uses.

Once again, INTENT is important. Hold clearly in the mind the purpose for which you intend to bathe and choose your essential oil very consciously, forming a mental image of the plant. Ask for the plant's help, as when choosing a massage oil.

Choose a quiet time when you will not be disturbed. Unless you live alone (or have two bathrooms!) make this a time when other members of the household are not likely to be clamouring for use of the bathroom. If your bathroom is brightly lit, as most are for functional reasons, consider using a candle instead of the normal light. When you are ready to get into the bath put a VERY FEW drops of your oil into the water; maybe three drops at the most. If you are using one of the flower absolutes (Jasmine, Neroli and Rose) or any other oil with very strong perfuming power, a single drop is enough. Some people like to add to the specialness of the occasion by floating a few flower petals on the water, but you may not always be able to obtain flowers of the same plant as your essential oil.

Now enter the bath and lie still for fifteen to twenty minutes, holding in your mind the result you wish to achieve by bathing in this way. Don't use this time for washing – if you need to clean physically, do it before you get into your special bath. When you get out of the bath, try to maintain the same quiet state for at least a little while. Wrap yourself in a towelling robe or big towel rather than rubbing dry vigorously.

A ritual bath can be a way to mark the change from mundane activities to special ones: for example, between doing the housework and offering a healing session to a friend, or between a hectic day at work and an evening meditation. Bathing in this way is particularly beautiful as a way of preparing to offer healing.

Such baths can be used to 'clear' after a bad experience – a row, a shock, an accident – or to clear the aura after being in crowded places such as shopping centres, public transport, etc., where you may be in proximity to energies you would not normally welcome into your personal space.

Another use is for self-healing: very valuable if you do not have access to a healer, aromatherapist or friend for massage or other form of healing.

Don't make a habit of ritual bathing – if you do much of

the value will be lost. After all, the idea of ritual implies something rather special. If you do it every day, it will just become your daily bath.

ROOM PERFUMING – BURNERS AND DIFFUSERS

The third method which we can borrow from conventional aromatherapy is room perfuming, using a burner or diffuser. This is perhaps the most subtle of the traditional methods, as it involves only the aroma of the plant, representing its energy in the most refined form. We experience the essential oil only in its gaseous state – the least solid form of physical matter.

It is also a very versatile method, for inhaling a vapour can be put to whatever purpose you wish, and can be applied to any and every essential oil (even those which cannot be used on the skin) depending on your wishes.

An essential oil burner is the easiest and cheapest equipment for room perfuming, although it does have the disadvantage of heating the essential oil which can change the aroma, particularly with the very delicate floral oils. 'Burner' is not a completely accurate description as the oil itself is not burnt, but heated by a nightlight so that it evaporates. Most burners are made of ceramics, and can be as plain or as fancy as you like. They have a space to hold a nightlight at the bottom, perforations of some kind to allow air to circulate and a dish at the top to hold the oil. Fill the dish with water and sprinkle a few drops of oil on the surface of the water: how many drops will depend on the size of the space you wish to perfume. Look for a burner with a big enough dish: too small and the water will evaporate long before the nightlight has finished burning, leaving the remaining oil to burn into a sticky, bad-smelling residue (which is very hard to clean off). Don't buy the metal burners which show up occasionally: contact with metal rapidly alters essential oils.

Apart from being cheap and simple, burners have two further advantages: they are silent and they produce a gentle light, very suitable for meditation.

To perfume a room about 3 metres square, float 4–6 drops of essential oil on the dish of water, more for a larger room. If you have a very large space to perfume, such as a hall used for workshops or a big meeting room used by a healing circle or meditation group, it is better to use two burners, maybe one at each end of the space, rather than put a great deal of essential oil in a single burner.

The alternative is an essential oil diffuser. These are small pieces of apparatus which use an electric pump to propel minuscule droplets of essential oil into the air.

The major advantages of diffusers is that they do not heat the essential oil, so there is no distortion of aroma. Another is that they can perfume a large space very quickly, which makes them more efficient than burners for workshops, etc. Their one drawback is that even the quietest make some noise which can be distracting during a healing session or meditation. You can use one to fill the space with the chosen oil before your activity begins and, if necessary, turn it on again briefly if there are breaks in the meeting.

The amount of essential oil released into the air with a diffuser is controlled by how long the apparatus is left running, rather than the amount of oil put in to start with.

Room perfuming has many applications and the results will depend largely on which essential oil is used.

As I have already suggested, one main use is to perfume a room that is going to be used for meditation, healing, etc. This closely resembles the traditional use of incense and, depending on which oils are used, can produce feelings of tranquillity, help deepen breathing and facilitate meditation in a number of ways which are covered in more detail in the chapter on Meditation.

An important use of burners or diffusers is in preparing a room that is sometimes used for meditation, healing, or similar activities, but the rest of the time for mundane purposes. This may be in your home, if you don't have enough space to set aside one room exclusively for such use, but is particularly important when using public spaces, hired halls, etc., for a healing circle, workshop or spiritual teaching.

The vibrations in such a space may not be at all suitable for your purpose, and you will need to clear any negative energy created by other users and create a more favourable environment for your subtle work. You may even need to clean the atmosphere at a purely physical level, to get rid of stale cigarette smoke, alcohol or cooking smells.

Burners can, of course, be an aid to individual meditation, just as much as for groups, in which case you should use only 2 or 3 drops of oil and put the burner fairly near where you will be sitting. An alternative for personal meditation is simply to inhale the oil from a handkerchief (see INHALING page 77).

Another use of room perfuming is to clear places where there has been some unpleasant event. Arguments, fights or any kind of trauma can leave very negative vibrations in the places where they took place and generally speaking, the more major the event, the longer the bad energy it gave rise to will remain. If you had a row with your spouse yesterday, burning a cleansing, cheerful oil will probably be enough to clear away the remaining negativity, but if your home is built on the site of an ancient battle, you would do well to use a burner or diffuser on a regular basis.

A less obvious use of vaporized oils is to facilitate all kinds of creativity. Writers, musicians, painters and crafts-people can benefit from using essential oils in their workplace. Certain oils are known to heighten creativity or activate the right (intuitive) side of the brain but the choice will depend very much on the individual, what sort of work they are doing and what they feel their needs to be at any particular moment. While Rose may be the oil that sparks off a flood of original ideas, Rosemary could help during the process of translating those ideas into concrete form.

Activating the right brain by use of oils is a valuable adjunct to creative visualization and guided imagery. Some people really find it quite difficult to 'see' images during such work and some Rosewood in a burner or a single drop of Rose or Helichrysum on a tissue may help the images to flow.

You can use a burner in combination with most of the other methods suggested in this book, vaporizing the same oil that you are using for a massage, for example, or one that compliments it in some way.

Massage, baths and burners/diffusers, then, are the main methods that can be simply adapted from traditional aromatherapy for more subtle uses, but there are some other ideas to be explored that are not part of the usual aroma-therapy repertoire.

AURIC MASSAGE

I have touched briefly on auric massage already, suggesting how it can be incorporated towards the end of an ordinary massage, but auric massage can also be used as a form of subtle healing in its own right. Dis-ease manifests in the subtle body before any physical symptoms are apparent, and the 'echoes' of illness and accidents can remain within a person's aura long after physical healing has taken place. The same is true of emotional trauma. In all these cases the vibrations within the aura are disturbed, and bringing appropriate essential oils into the aura helps to restore harmony.

Auric massage influences at very refined levels, and even if there is no negativity that may be connected with trauma or dis-ease, this way of working harmonizes the aura and helps to repair 'holes' through which energy can leak.

To give an auric massage, you do not need to mix essential oil in a carrier (unless you plan to include some physical massage in the same session). Simply put a drop of the chosen oil(s) on your hands before you begin. If you feel it is necessary, take another drop at intervals during the session. The person receiving the massage does not need to undress. Before you put any oil on your hands, rest your hands gently on your friend's head for a few moments to establish contact. Lift your hands away very slowly, trying to feel the connection that remains between your friend's head and your hands even though they are no longer touching. Now move your hands about above your friend's body to find how far out you can still feel this connection. It will probably vary from one part of the body to another, sometimes quite noticeably.

Now put a drop of oil on your hands and begin to make gentle stroking movements at the level where you feel the energy connection strongly, varying this whenever appropriate. You will probably find places where the energy feels different, lacking, disturbed or broken. Differences in the way the aura feels can be due to physical illness, emotional trauma, grief, depression, drugs (whether prescribed or otherwise) and even such things as cigarettes and coffee. One spiritual teacher says that a single cigarette blackens the aura for an hour. You don't need to know what is causing a change in the way your friend's aura feels in order to heal it: just respond to these changes intuitively by changing your strokes. You might want to make some short, brisk movements, vary the direction of your stroking, work in circles or hold your hands still for a while, but whatever you do, follow your intuition. If you enjoy working with crystals, you might like to use one to carry out an auric massage. An egg-shaped crystal, a sphere, or the long, flat side of a pointed crystal are all suitable for massaging the aura.

End the session in the way I have already described in relation to conventional massage, and stay with your friend until you are certain that he or she is fully awake (people quite often fall asleep during auric massage) and focused on the immediate surroundings. It may be appropriate to talk at this point but some people may wish to be quiet.

Similarly, some therapists like to maintain silence during the auric massage, some appreciate feedback from the recipient and some may wish to give some gentle suggestions, such as asking the recipient to focus attention on a particular area.

WORKING WITH CRYSTALS

Using essential oils and crystals together in healing is a major branch of subtle aromatherapy and you will find a whole chapter devoted to this area.

WORKING WITH CHAKRA ENERGY

The same is true of working with the Chakras, and in fact there is a great deal of overlap here, as crystals are used extensively with the essential oils in Chakra healing and balancing. Again, you will find a chapter dealing with Chakra work in detail.

ANOINTING

Putting oil directly on the body is a very ancient practice, common to many religions and spiritual traditions. It survives, for example, in the coronation ceremony which indicates one of its uses, that is, to mark one person as special. As well as showing her love and devotion, this is what Mary Magdalene was doing when she anointed Christ's head and feet with oil of Spikenard and other costly aromatics. It was also she who anointed His body with sweet spices, Myrrh and Frankincense after it was taken down from the cross. A king, priest or shaman may be anointed with oil to signify their particular office, and there is often special significance in the oils chosen. Priests of many different religions anoint the sick with oils when death seems to be imminent, and this practice is known to bring great serenity to the dying.

Anointing can also be used as a form of protection, by putting a few drops of oil such as Rosemary, Juniper or Vetivert on the body before going into a threatening situation or a place where the prevailing energy is unpleasant. Some therapists practise self-anointing before working with clients, both to invoke healing energies and to protect themselves from any negativity they might otherwise attract from the client.

Anointing oils are usually applied to areas of the body that hold some symbolic significance, such as the head, breast, hands or feet, and in fact all these places correspond to various chakras. If anointing is being done for protection, the oil should be applied to the Solar Plexus area with anticlockwise movements.

Anointing is a particularly appropriate way of working with people who are terminally ill. It can evoke a deep spiritual response at a time when physical aromatherapy treatment is no longer relevant.

INHALING

Simply smelling an essential oil can dramatically change our state of awareness, and is often the best way to use essential oils to assist visualization or strengthen affirmations.

Sniffing the oil direct from the bottle is often overpowering, so just putting a drop on a tissue, cotton bud or handkerchief is better. A single drop is all that is needed: inhale it deeply before beginning a visualization, meditation or affirmation.

Inhale deeply again at the end to anchor the experience.

SMOKING, SMUDGING AND INCENSE

Although none of these is strictly speaking aromatherapy (as essential oils are not used) I have included them because they work on exactly the same principle of inhaling an aromatic vapour to influence the psyche and can be effectively used instead of essential oils in some situations.

Smoking involves burning dried twigs, leaves or wood from aromatic plants to produce a perfumed smoke. Woody shrubs such as Juniper and Rosemary are the most suitable.

The use of aromatic smoke for healing, magic, ritual and to achieve trance states predates written history by many thousands of years. Our earliest ancestors probably stumbled upon the effects of scented smoke accidentally when using branches from aromatic trees or shrubs as firewood. Fossilised pollens and ashes found during archaeological digs show that people were using aromatic plants more than 60,000 years ago, and probably long before that. Smoking was widely practised in mediaeval Europe to 'drive out evil spirits' and we can still use it to clear houses of any bad energy, as described under 'Room Perfuming'. It is less suitable for perfuming rooms before meditation, etc., simply because the smoke can be irritating and possibly provoke an outbreak of coughing.

If you have an open fire, just throw a few sprigs of your chosen plant onto hot coals or logs. If not, you could burn some sprigs in any fire-proof container, though you might need some other inflammable material to get the dried plant material to burn.

Smudging is the form of smoking used by Native Americans, who usually use dried Cedar, Sage and Sweetgrass bound together to make a smudge-stick. Some tribes at the present time add Lavender, but this is a relatively recent introduction as Lavender is not native to the American continent. (The Cedar and Sage used are not the European varieties – see notes under the entries for these oils.) Cedar is used for balance and to get rid of nightmares. Sage is for purification and Sweetgrass brings in beauty, or as so poetically phrased by the original holders of this tradition 'Sage is to banish, Cedar to balance and Sweetgrass to bless'. These herbs may be burnt in sweatlodges, at ceremonial sites or near a person who needs healing, protection or purifying. Sweetgrass, known as 'the hair of Grandmother Earth' is sometimes plaited and burnt on its own.

Smudging is increasingly used by people other than Native Americans for similar purposes, especially by those interested in earthlore and shamanistic traditions.

The herbs are burnt traditionally in an abalone shell or a fireproof pottery dish. Once you have ignited the herbs, wave a big feather over the shell or dish to waft the smoke in the direction you want it to go. If you are cleansing or dedicating a space, you should send smoke to each of the four directions, North, South, East and West and, if you feel it is appropriate, call on the energies of the Earth, Moon, Sun, animals, plants and minerals to assist. To smudge an individual, walk round the person slowly, fanning the smoke towards them with the feather, starting near the ground and ending just above the head. The feather should traditionally be from an eagle, but I use a goose-feather which has a long tradition of use in Celtic cultures.

Incenses are compounded mainly of aromatic gums and resins to produce scented smoke and, of course, are used in the major religions of both East and West as well as other spiritual traditions. Incense subtly changes the awareness, in much the same way as some essential oils, making it easier to enter a meditative or devotional state of mind. It is also used to cleanse, purify and invoke blessing like the other forms of smoking.

Incense sold in the form of joss-sticks is usually of very poor quality and may contain adulterants. The actual perfuming ingredients in cheaper joss-sticks are often synthetic, so they are no use at all for subtle energy purposes. Buy loose incense and some charcoal discs on which to ignite it.

There are many different incenses available. Some of them are made from the same resins as the corresponding essential oils (Myrrh, Frankincense, Benzoin, etc.) so you can deduce their properties. Others will have names that suggest their use. If you are not sure whether a particular incense is for meditation, purification, etc., ask the supplier, who ought to know.

Although these notes cover all the ways of using essential oils and other materials suggested in this book, they should not be thought of as definitive. As I suggested at the beginning of this chapter, feel free to adapt, discard or invent. These are the methods that have worked for me, my friends and colleagues but only experiment will show whether they feel right for you. If not, there are no 'rules' to prevent you from creating new ways of working. That's how knowledge is expanded.

The only thing that matters is that the essential oils are used to benefit humanity.

CHAPTER 7

Dowsing and Aromatherapy

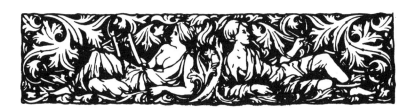

A pendulum is a very useful instrument for anybody working with subtle energies: simple to use, versatile in its applications, small, portable and available for use anywhere.

How does a pendulum work? I believe it amplifies the intuition of the user. A pendulum does not know anything or possess supernatural properties. Rather, it helps the user to tap into his or her unconscious mind and perhaps the collective unconscious as well.

Anybody can use a pendulum. There is no mystery involved and no special skill needed. Simply trust in the fact that a pendulum can be of use to you, and it will.

Many readers will already be familiar with the use of a pendulum – dowsing – but for those who are not I will briefly outline the system before going on to discuss how it may be applied in subtle aromatherapy.

A pendulum is a small object on the end of a cord, like a plumber's bob-line. Anything will do so long as it is heavy enough to make the cord hang vertically when still. Wedding rings are often used and I have improvised an effective pendulum from a brass button and a piece of string. Ready made pendulums may be made from wood, metal, crystal and other materials and in a variety of shapes, such as pear or tear-drop shape, conical or like an inverted onion though for sensitive work the best shapes are those that are pointed towards the bottom. If you think you will work regularly with a pendulum it is worth seeking out one that feels exactly right for you. It should feel comfortable in your hand and you should find its appearance pleasing to your eye. Once you have made your choice, remember to keep your pendulum in a carrying pouch or wrap it in a handkerchief or cloth when you are not using it.

A pendulum is most often used to answer questions, though there are other uses which I shall touch on later. The questions must be capable of being answered with a yes or no and the answer is deduced from the direction in which the pendulum swings. For example, the pendulum may swing in a clockwise circle for yes and anticlockwise for no, or it may swing backwards and forwards for one and from side to side for the other, or again it may show a circular swing for one answer and a straight one for the other. This will vary from one person to another and from one pendulum to another. Because a pendulum swings in a particular way for your friend, it does not necessarily mean that it will swing the same way for you, so the first thing you need to do when working with a pendulum that is new to you is to establish how it is going to swing when you use it.

To do this, hold the string or chain between your thumb and forefinger so that the pendulum hangs vertically and still from your hand. It often helps to rest your elbow on a table or other flat surface and some people also like to support their wrist with the other hand to keep the working hand quite still. Your hand should not move at all: when you begin working with the pendulum it will swing of its own accord without any movement from your hand. You may like to try the pendulum in your right hand and then your left, to find out which works best for you.

Start by finding out the response for a 'yes' answer. You can do this either by asking directly 'Please show me the direction for yes', or by asking a question to which you know the answer is positive. For example, you might hold the pendulum over a bottle of Lavender oil, and ask 'Is this a bottle of Lavender oil?'. Whichever swing you then observe will be the response for 'yes'. Next, you repeat the process to find the direction of swing for 'no'. You do not need to ask these questions out loud, though it is perfectly acceptable to do so if that is the way you would like to work. It is quite sufficient to phrase the questions mentally.

Once you have established the directions in which your pendulum swings for the two possible answers, you will usually find that other pendulums swing in the same directions when you use them (even though they may show a different swing when used by somebody else). This is not infallible, though, so you do need to go through this procedure again each time you work with a new pendulum. You can be reasonably sure that once you have established the directions with a particular pendulum, they will be constant, but even this is not quite certain. I used to think that, once established, the swing of a particular pendulum for a particular user was unchanging, until I acquired a very heavy brass pendulum which changes its swing from time to time, so when working with that particular instrument I have to establish the swing afresh at the beginning of each session. This is, however, very unusual.

As well as the direction of swing, you may observe differences in the speed and the amplitude of the swing and in some applications these can be used as a gauge of emphasis. For example: you might try using your pendulum to establish whether certain foods have been organically grown. You could ask the question 'Are there any chemical residues in this food?' and repeat it for each item in turn. A very large and/or rapid 'Yes' swing would indicate a high level of chemical residues, while a smaller one would suggest a lesser degree of contamination.

If you are new to dowsing, practise using your pendulum often until you feel confident about using it.

When we come to applying dowsing to subtle aromatherapy there are several areas in which it can be invaluable. One of these is determining whether an essential oil is pure, unadulterated, authentic, etc. While these factors are important in conventional aromatherapy, they are perhaps even more so when working at a subtle level, as the smallest departure from purity will, of course, change the vibration of the oil. Although I buy all my oils from a tiny handful of suppliers who I trust, I will still apply the pendulum test from time to time to newly-acquired oils. Because my suppliers are meticulous about their sources, I am seldom disappointed but it is really imperative to test oils in this way if the supplier is not known to you. Begin with the question 'Is this oil from the plant species named on the label?' or, if you feel the labelling is inadequate, specify the species from which the authentic oil should be derived. This initial question can be vital, especially if you are dealing with an oil such as Melissa, where other lemon-scented oils are often substituted because of its cost and scarcity. In this particular instance, if the oil is not Melissa, it will be totally useless for work at a subtle level that specifically needs the vibrational energy of Melissa.

Once you have established that your oil is indeed what it claims to be, you can continue with such questions as 'Are there any chemical residues in this oil?', 'Are there any other adulterants in this oil?', 'Is this oil diluted?' etc. Ideally, the answer to each one of these questions should be 'No'. If the pendulum indicates that there is any kind of adulteration, you could go on and ask whether there were synthetic substances added to the oil or whether it had been mixed with essential oils, or fractions of essential oils, from plants other than the one required, though such information would only be for your own interest, since an oil with any kind of extraneous material in it is useless for subtle work.

The second area in which dowsing can be extremely helpful is in deciding which oil is likely to be most helpful for the use you have in mind at any particular time. Some aromatherapists dowse to find the best oil, or blend of oils to use for a client when practising conventional aromatherapy, although the trained therapist really should know the properties and uses of each oil so intimately that the choice for each client presents itself without difficulty. In subtle aromatherapy, though, the established properties and uses of an oil may not always be the best guide to its subtle use. Indeed, what we know intellectually about an oil may sometimes get in the way of our intuitive response to that oil.

Even the few guidelines that exist as to the subtle action of oils can only be general pointers because we are dealing with very fine vibrations, and with the reaction between the vibrations of a plant and its essential oil, and the vibrations of the individual or group using it. You may also find that there are a number of oils that are each, theoretically, capable of the effect you are seeking: dowsing can help you find the most appropriate.

To find the best oil for your purpose, it would be wasteful of time and energy to dowse through every oil you own, unless your collection is very small. From your previous experience with the oils, or from the guidelines in this or other books, select those that seem most likely to be helpful, and then dowse to make your final selection from among them. Alternatively, you might make your initial selection by dividing your collection into three or four sections, and dowsing with the question 'Is the oil I am seeking among this group of bottles?'. My own oil collection is housed in four boxes, so I use the question 'Is the oil I need in this box?'. This can sometimes save a lot of time by reducing the number of bottles you need to test. However, if the final choice is to be a blend, it can equally well be that the various components are spread among your collection in which case this approach will not help, and you will get a 'Yes' for every box, or group of bottles.

Having selected your small group of possible oils, you can then dowse with a question such as 'Which of these oils will help ... at this time?' (inserting the name of the person to be helped). Or you might want to ask 'Which of these oils will best enhance our group meditation today?'. You will note that in each of these questions the present time is mentioned: this is important, because the right choice of oil might be different tomorrow or next week even though the same people are involved. This is, of course, just as true in conventional aromatherapy, so if you are progressing from conventional to more subtle work the principle will already be familiar.

Place your bottles far enough apart for the pendulum to swing clearly above each one in turn without being influenced by the adjacent bottles. If you place them too close together you may get an inconclusive result. When dowsing in this particular context you may find that the pendulum gives a 'no' response over any oil that is not particularly appropriate for your immediate use, or it may simply not move at all. The response to oils that are likely to be helpful may vary in speed or size of the swing, which might enable you to select a single oil as the best choice.

If not, you can remove all the oils to which there was a negative response and proceed with the rest. If these do not number more than three or four, you might like simply to make them into a blend, or you may dowse again asking whether a blend would be best. If, as a result of dowsing or your own decision, you do not want to make a blend, you can dowse further, using the question 'Which single oil from among these three (or however many) is the one I should use?'.

To dowse in this way may seem long and complicated in the telling, but in fact takes very little time to do and of course the more you dowse and the more confident and familiar you become with the process, the faster you will be able to carry it out.

When I dowse for oils in this manner, I turn the bottles so that the labels are facing away from me, so that I am not in any way influenced by what I know intellectually about each oil. In this way I can be more sure of reacting intuitively to the energy or vibration of the oil.

This particular form of dowsing is especially valuable if you want to select an oil, or oils, for your personal use at a subtle level.

When you are working with another person or a group, there is always an interplay between your own energy and that of the other person or people involved. If you are sensitive and receptive to other people you will seldom have difficulty in sensing the needs of anybody you are trying to help. How much harder it is to know our own needs, especially at the most subtle levels! If you have access to another aromatherapist or healer I think it is always preferable to seek their help rather than prescribe for oneself. However, there are inevitably times when we need help, and outside help is not at hand, and at such times the pendulum can almost take the place of another person's input.

When you need to choose an oil for your personal use, it is worth spending a few minutes beforehand trying to clear your mind of all preconceptions about your present state and which oils may be appropriate to it. Develop an attitude of trust in your higher self and its ability to guide your choice. In this way you are most likely to arrive at the most appropriate oil, whether you dowse or choose by some other means. When the choice is made, do not let your intellectual knowledge about the properties of the oil, whether subtle or physical, make you question that choice or change it unless there is a compelling reason to do so, such as a physical condition that rules out the use of that oil (pregnancy, high blood pressure, epilepsy, etc.). However, I have never known an oil to be chosen in this way for subtle use that would be physically damaging to the user.

It is usually simpler to decide on the best method of use; bathing, anointing, vaporizing, etc., than on the oil or blend to use, but if you are in any doubt, you can always dowse for the best method by asking such questions as 'Would

auric massage be the best way to use this oil for . . . . . today?'
(putting in the name of the person to be helped).

Occasionally, it can be beneficial to dowse to find whether
the proposed time for a healing, meditation, etc., is the most
appropriate. The time of day, the moon's phases, planetary
influences and the ever-changing energies of the people
involved – both the healer and the person needed healing –
can influence the outcome. Most people contemplating
subtle work of this kind will instinctively know if the time is
wrong, but if unsure at any time, use the pendulum to judge.

Testing oils and choosing oils, methods and times all
involve using the pendulum to answer questions but it can
be put to one or two other uses in subtle aromatherapy. In
particular, a pendulum can be used when working with the
chakras, to assess the energy state of each chakra before and
after a healing, and this will be described fully in the chapter
on the chakras. Some healers use a pendulum made of
quartz, amethyst or other crystals as a direct healing tool,
and again this will be covered in the appropriate part of this
book.

You can use a pendulum to locate ley-lines and other
manifestations of earth-energy, both beneficial and harmful.
This can be very valuable in healing as there is an increasing
body of evidence that some people become ill, recover very
slowly or do not respond to treatment because they are
living on a ley-line crossover point, or sleeping in a part of
their home that is affected by some negative earth-energy.
The term geopathic stress is used to describe such influences
on our wellbeing. If anybody you know – a client, relative or
friend or indeed yourself – has become ill since moving house,
or feels abnormally tired for no discernable reason, heals
slowly or fails to recover from any condition in spite of
treatment, etc., or if you know of a house where a succession
of inhabitants have become ill one after another, you would
do well to investigate the possibility of geopathic stress.

Dowsing can be used to locate the negative energy sources that cause geopathic stress, either on a map or at the actual location. Dowsing a map can save a lot of time at an actual site.

To dowse a map, it is helpful to have a pendulum with a fine point, and to have as large-scale map as you can obtain. It might be helpful to get a small section of a map enlarged if you are trying to pinpoint some influence within a relatively small area. Before starting, ask your pendulum to show you how it will swing when the particular feature you are looking for is located. Most often, this will be a circular swing over the map point. If the energy at that point is very powerful, it will cause a correspondingly large swing of the pendulum, and on small-scale maps this can be very confusing as the pendulum circle can cover an area that represents perhaps several miles. However, with a suitable pendulum, a big enough map and some practice this is not difficult.

To dowse at an actual location, some people prefer to use dowsing rods, but I have used a pendulum equally successfully. Be clear about what you are looking for, and ask the pendulum to move when it is located. The pendulum will remain inert until you approach the source of negative energy, or the ley-line, or whatever you are looking for and start moving as soon as you get close enough to the energy source. It will stop moving when you move out of that field of energy again, so you can pinpoint quite precise areas of energy.

If you feel unsure about dowsing for negative or positive earth energies, you might consider employing an experienced dowser to do this for you.

The information thus gained can be instrumental in healing, as it is sometimes only necessary to move a bed a few feet, or a desk or chair where an ailing person spends a lot of time, for the healing processes to be set in motion.

Where it is impossible to make a simple adjustment of that kind, for example, if a whole room, or a whole house is affected, it is possible to buy instruments that counteract the adverse effects of geopathic stress. Depending on the source of the problem you may be able to use crystals and essential oils to heal the environment and we will look at some of the ways of doing this in another chapter.

Of course, you can equally well dowse to find areas of positive, life-giving energy and consciously use them for healing, meditation, to locate your bed, desk, etc. as a way of increasing your physical health and subtle energies.

If you would rather use divining rods than a pendulum for this kind of work, they are very easy to make. You need two wire coathangers and two ballpoint or felt-tip pens that have finished their useful life. Cut each coathanger so that you have a piece of wire about 20 inches long and bend it at right angles so that you have a short side about 8 inches in length and a long side of about 12 inches. Remove the inside from each pen, so that you are left with two plastic tubes. Drop the short end of each piece of wire into one of the plastic tubes. Hold a tube in each hand, with the wire pointing straight forward. When you approach the energy-source you are looking for, the wire rods will swing apart and point out to the sides and as you move away from it they will swing back to their original position. Water diviners have dowsed in this way for hidden water sources since time immemorial.

The art of dowsing to select the most suitable place to live in relation to the surrounding earth energy is known as geomancy and was very widely used in earlier times, especially in China. No building would be commenced until the site had been dowsed to ascertain that the prevailing energy would be beneficial to the future inhabitants, and to determine the best alignment of the building.

If you locate an area of negative energy in a house, you

will then need to find out what kind of energy is involved, so that you can decide whether to use essential oils, meditation, crystals to clear or negate it, or whether it would be more effective to buy a small device known as a RadiTech that plugs into an electrical circuit to do this. As a general guide, if the cause is a specific physical one, such as underground water, mineral deposits or harmful earth rays, a RadiTech would probably be more effective. If you are dealing with negative energies that cannot be traced to any physical cause, meditation with essential oils, or crystals, or any combination of these three will probably be more appropriate. (I am not referring here to 'ghosts' or exorcism. That is something else entirely and not for the subtle aromatherapist to meddle with.)

To discover whether areas of negative energy in a house are the result of actual geophysical features, or perhaps negative thought-forms lingering from past events or earlier occupants, you may need to ask the pendulum some supplementary questions. You might phrase a question such as 'Is this area of negativity due to physical influences?' and if you obtain a 'yes' answer, you might then ask if an electrical device would be the best solution. If you get a 'no' answer to the first question, you could ask 'Is this area of bad energy caused by negative thought-forms?'. If the answer to this is 'yes' you could ask whether essential oils, meditation or crystals would help to clear it. (Remember that this would require three separate questions, as the pendulum can only give 'yes' or 'no' answers.)

A pendulum can be used for other purposes outside the scope of this book, such as identifying food allergies, locating lost objects or finding sources of water and so forth. You will probably be able to think of other applications.

The only valid criterion is that you use the pendulum with the genuine intention of obtaining information that will enable you to heal, to help or to be of service in some other way. If you use a pendulum to ask questions frivolously, or to try to obtain information that should not, by rights, be made available to you, in all probability you will get no response. The pendulum is not a toy, and should be used responsibly and ethically, just as you would use essential oils.

CHAPTER 8

Chakra
Energies and
Essential Oils

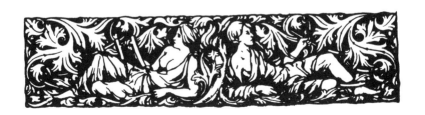

W orking with essential oils that influence the chakras or energy centres of the body, is one of the major fields of Subtle Aromatherapy and it is also one of the easiest to understand and put into practice for those who are new to subtle healing work. The underlying theory of chakra energy has been outlined in the chapter on 'Subtle Anatomy' (although I am sure many readers are already familiar with this in more detail than is possible here) and in order to understand the relationship between chakra energy and essential oils we need now to explore the individual chakras.

As you read the following outline of the nature of each of the major chakras, see whether any essential oils suggest themselves to you. I will, of course, discuss the relationship of essential oils and the individual chakras a little further on, but your learning will go deeper if you start making such connections for yourself. Don't think too hard! Just be open to any spontaneous thoughts or feelings about appropriate oils that may arise.

THE SEVEN MAJOR CHAKRAS
The Base Chakra

The Base Chakra is usually described as being situated at the base of the spine, though some teachers describe its location as being the perineum (the muscular area between the anus and the genitals) and I find the latter more convincing. The energy-colour of this chakra is red, and its sound is LAM.

This chakra is connected with the element Earth, the most solid of the elements, and its associated shape is the square. (This is not the shape of the chakra itself, but a shape that traditionally represents the Earth element.) It helps even more to understand the character of Base Chakra energy if you think of a cube, the three-dimensional form of a square. A cube is the most solid of all geometrical shapes: it sits solidly on the Earth, difficult to displace. The vibration of this chakra is the slowest of the seven.

The focus of the Base Chakra is physical survival, and basic necessities such as food, drink and sleep. Its Sanskrit name means 'The Foundation' and this chakra supports all higher activities. It is also the point at which we are grounded, or connected to Earth energies. Think of a person sitting to meditate in the traditional lotus posture, or simply cross-legged: the perineum will be touching the Earth. Physical analogies such as this can tell us much about the vibrational nature of each chakra. If a person is lacking in physical energy, the Base Chakra will probably be depleted or blocked. This is also true if somebody feels ungrounded, 'spacey' or 'lives in their head'.

The Sacral Chakra

This chakra is located at the level of the sacrum (a large triangular bone in the lower spine) corresponding to a point slightly below the navel. Its energy-colour is orange and its sound is VAM.

The Sacral Chakra relates to the element Water, and its associated shape is the circle or sphere. A sphere is far less stable than cube but equally, it is freer. A sphere can move in all directions, like the element is symbolises – Water.

This is the centre of sexual and creative energy. It is connected also with the watery elements within the body. In the literal sense, seminal fluid, menstrual flow, urine and the fluids in the intestines are all influenced by the Sacral Chakra. Less literally, we can think of this energy in relation to the 'flow' of creativity and the movement of 'emotional tides'. All creative impulses originate here, whether they be the making of a new life, a poem or a painting. Too much or too little energy in the chakra may relate to sexual difficulties or more general problems in relating, but equally to creative difficulties, such as writer's block.

The Solar Plexus Chakra

The Solar Plexus Chakra is located at approximately waist level. Its energy-colour is yellow, and its sound is RAM.

It relates to the element of Fire, and its shape is the triangle or prism. The prism leads the eye upwards towards it apex, and denotes the upward-moving nature of Fire. A prism also channels light, which is a part of the Fire element. Without Fire (i.e. the Sun) there would be no light.

This is where we relate to the outer world. Shock and stressful events affect this chakra more directly than the others. It is the centre of our will, but also where we connect with the Divine Will. If the individual will is in harmony with the Divine, the Solar Plexus Chakra will generally be in balance. People who are under a lot of stress will almost always show some imbalance in this chakra. The Fire element is concerned with digestion, with the stomach and the liver – consider how many stressed people suffer from digestive problems!

The Heart Chakra

The Heart Chakra is situated level with the physical heart. Its sound is YAM, and its energy-colour is usually described as green, in keeping with the spectrum order of colours shown in the seven major chakras. However, there is a very strong connection between Heart Chakra energy and the colour pink, and some sources show this chakra as having green at the centre surrounded by pink, which is how I always envisage it.

The ruling element is Air, and the shape a crescent or saucer-like shape. This symbolizes the completely free nature of the Air element: a dish is open – you can't keep Air enclosed within it.

The Heart Chakra is concerned with love (you guessed!). This may be love for another individual, the Unconditional Love that connects us to the whole Universe or devotional love for a Deity. It is also the point of connection between the upper and lower chakras. The three lower chakras, Base, Sacral and Solar Plexus, are primarily concerned with our experience of the physical world: the three upper chakras, Throat, Brow and Crown are concerned with mental and spiritual experiences. The Heart Chakra links and balances these opposites. If energy does not flow freely between Solar Plexus and Heart, or between Heart and Throat, this link is incomplete and there will be an imbalance somewhere in the energy system.

The Heart Chakra can also be thought of as a link between body and spirit, through its connection with the Air element. Literally, the air entering and leaving our lungs (which lie close to the Heart Chakra) maintains life. Without air, life ceases and the spirit and physical body are separated. Symbolically, air or, more specifically, the breath connects our limited human selves to our higher selves and to more spiritual planes of being. Breathing is central to most forms of meditation, and so helps us to achieve that connection. Consider for a moment the literal and symbolic meanings of the words 'aspire', 'inspire' and 'expire'.

The Throat Chakra

This is situated at the base of the throat. Its energy-colour is blue and its sound is HAM.

Its element is Ether, within which all the other elements are present in a pure and rarefied state (you could say they were etherial) and the shape is a star. A star radiates its energy outwards, which is a function of the Throat Chakra.

The Throat Chakra is concerned with expression, in particular with giving outward expression to the truths understood by the Heart Chakra and the creative impulses of the Sacral Chakra. The vehicle of this expression may be the voice (this chakra being in the region of the vocal cords) but it may equally well be any of the arts. At a very subtle level the Throat Chakra relates to spiritual teaching, and certain teachers have highly refined energy in this Chakra. People who find it hard to communicate, or who are denied the opportunity to give outer expression to their creativity will usually have some blockage or imbalance at the Throat Chakra. This chakra will also show much imbalance in individuals who are not living their truth.

The Brow Chakra

This is situated in the centre of the forehead, at the location of the third eye. There is no element associated with the Brow Chakra, as its vibrations are higher than any physical manifestation. Its colour is indigo and its sound is AUM.

The Brow Chakra is associated with intellect and understanding. This may be the rational intellect but in some individuals concerns occult knowledge, clairvoyance or channelling which is symbolised by the idea of the third eye. Understanding also implies an understanding of moral issues and the lessons to be learnt in this life. Working with this chakra will usually benefit anybody who is woolly-minded, as well as those who are engaged in much intellectual effort. The energy is likely to be distorted in those who close their eyes to the lessons implicit in a human incarnation.

The Crown Chakra

The Crown Chakra, or Thousand-Petalled Lotus, is located at the top of the head. Its centre is at the point where the plates of the skull meet (the fontanelle or soft spot on a baby's head) but its petals extend to cover the whole crown of the head.

Like the Brow Chakra, the Crown is not linked to any element, for its vibration is pure spirit. Its colour is usually described as violet, but you should think of this as a transparent, luminous amethyst shade. The thousand petals are often depicted in rainbow colours, as this is the summing-up of all the chakras and contains within it all their colours. Its sound is the same as that of the Brow Chakra – the cosmic sound of AUM – but resonating at a higher octave.

The Crown Chakra embodies our spirituality. It is the seat of the Guru Within. It enables us to express our highest wisdom, and to be open to the ultimate Wisdom. There is often significant opening of the Crown Chakra during meditation, contemplation and prayer and individuals who are highly evolved at a spiritual level will have this chakra fully open all the time. In Christian art, the haloes surrounding the heads of Christ and his saints are an attempt by the artist to depict this outpouring of spiritual energy. In Eastern art, the Buddha, bodhisatvas and other highly evolved beings are often shown with a 'topknot' or crown protuberance which is meant to denote a highly developed Crown Chakra.

You may find some blocking in this chakra in people who are unwilling or afraid to open to their own spiritual potential. The energy will probably be rather deficient in people who are very attached to the material aspects of human life.

Above the Crown chakra, there are others, of an increasingly refined nature, situated in the aura beyond the crown of the head.

Most healers include the Eighth Chakra, and you will probably be able to sense where this is with most people, but you can, if you wish, take into consideration another four chakras beyond that, i.e. up to the Twelfth Chakra.

NOTE: THE SOUNDS OF THE CHAKRAS. The sounds printed above with each chakra should be pronounced as if the 'M' was a nasal 'N', so LAM sounds more or less like 'Long'. The initial consonant of each sound is emphasised, and the 'ng'-like sound at the end allowed to continue in the nose as if you were humming. If you want to chant these sounds, they are usually all sounded on the name note, but if it feels more appropriate to you, there is no reason why you should not move up through a rising scale. Some people prefer to simply chant AUM (OM) for all the chakras, starting with the lowest note they can make for the Base Chakra and moving up a scale. If neither of these possibilities feels right to you, if they do not resonate with the energy you feel in your own centres, then explore the world of sounds until you discover what feels exactly right for you.

SECONDARY CHAKRAS

I mentioned earlier the secondary chakras in the hands, feet and knees, and these are deserving of some consideration here. Those located at the knee are concerned with the business of moving forward through this life's journey, just as the physical knees lead the body forwards when walking. Some work around this area will often help people who feel 'stuck' or unsure of their path.

The chakras in the feet are another point of connection with the Earth. Work on the feet, as well as the area of the Base Chakra, for people who seem ungrounded, also at the end of auric massage which can often leave the receiver feeling very detached and 'floaty'.

The chakras in the hands are located at the centre of the palm, and correspond to the point where many therapists can feel healing energy most strongly. If you tried some of the energy-exchange exercises in 'The Role of the Healer' you may have experienced heat, tingling or a sensation like the pull of a magnet in this part of your hand. You may have felt such sensations at the fingertips instead or as well as the palm, and there are smaller chakras at the tips of the fingers, too.

There are many more aspects to the study of the chakras, though there is not room to explore all of them here. If this area of work appeals to you, I strongly advise reading a lot more, and would like to suggest 'Chakras, Energy Centres of Transformation' by Harish Johari as one of the best sources of information.

ESSENTIAL OILS AND CHAKRAS

Now that you have at least an outline idea of the major chakras we can begin to explore the relationship between chakras and essential oils.

No two 'experts' seem to agree completely on which oils work with which chakras. I think this is partly because we are dealing here with elusive and ever-changing energies, and partly because various people when compiling lists or charts of chakras and oils, may not have had the same purpose or end-result in mind. Essential oils can influence chakra energy in a variety of ways: energising, calming, reinforcing the activity of one specific chakra, or balancing all of them, and so forth. So, what we really need to be looking for is a number of different oils for each chakra, which we can use according to individual needs.

Correlations between essential oils and chakras can be arrived at in various ways. Sometimes colour is the link, and this may be the colour of the actual oil, the colour of the flower it came from or the 'colour' of the aroma (as in 'a green smell' or a 'dark brown smell'). Sometimes the part of the plant from which the oil is derived, or even the type of plant, its shape, size, etc. may lead you to make a connection with a particular chakra. Much of the information in 'The

Healing Energies of Plants' is very relevant here. You might perceive a connection by applying what you know about the oil's subtle properties, you could dowse, you might wish to meditate on each chakra in turn or you may simply feel intuitively that an oil is right. All of these paths are valid, and most therapists will use several of them.

MAJOR OILS FOR THE MAJOR CHAKRAS
The Base Chakra

Essential oils that resonate at the Base Chakra are generally those which are grounding, strengthening and centring. Mostly, they will be oils that are traditionally classed as Base Notes in perfumery and several are brown or reddish in colour. Among these we find Myrrh, a reddish-brown, dark, hot and smoky in character, which has an energising effect of greatest value when the Base Chakra energy is depleted. Patchouli, also dark brown, with a deep, extremely long-lasting, earthy aroma, is very grounding in effect, and helps those who tend to live in their heads. Vetivert is yet another deep brown oil, extracted from the roots of a fragrant grass, and is strongly grounding, but it also has a balancing and protective character. As well as its value at the Base Chakra level, it balances the energy through all the chakras, and has a special relevance for the Solar Plexus as a protector. Frankincense and Rosewood are also linking oils, resonating with both the Base and the Crown Chakra. Elemi is closely related to Frankincense and very similar in character, helping us to understand the unity of body and spirit.

The Sacral Chakra

The oils that have greatest affinity for this chakra are usually less dense in character than Base Chakra oils and include many of the aphrodisiac oils. Among these, Jasmine is the supreme example, deeply sensual and warming in nature. Jasmine also resonates at the Heart and Crown Chakras, linking the centres of love and spirituality to the sexual centre. Rose, equally complex though softer in its character, also works at all these levels. At the Sacral Chakra, Rose connects with sexual and reproductive energy and also with the fount of creativity, as expressed in all the arts or simply as a great love of beauty. (Jasmine, too, is thought to favour artistic development and love of the arts.) Sandalwood is another oil for the Sacral Chakra, and this, too, also resonates in its higher frequencies with the Crown Chakra.

The Solar Plexus Chakra

Two very important oils for the Solar Plexus are Juniper and Vetivert (and it is worth noticing that both these would be passed over if one relied solely on colour relationships in seeking the most appropriate oils for each chakra). Vetivert is a protector and balancer, as we saw already with the Base Chakra and Juniper is a cleanser. If you know that you are going into a crowded public place, or any situation that makes you feel uncomfortable or fearful, it is good to anoint the Solar Plexus chakra with a drop or two of Vetivert beforehand, always applying it in an anti-clockwise direction. Should you find yourself in such a situation without having been protected beforehand, and if you feel that other peoples' energies have been intruding on you, Juniper will quickly help to clear them.

The Heart Chakra

This is the point of balance between the upper and lower chakras, and the centre of love, and a number of very beautiful oils are associated with this chakra. The one that comes first to everybody's mind is Rose, which is truly the essence of love. Rose intensifies the loving energy of the Heart Chakra, and is deeply healing when this chakra is closed through grief. We associate Rose with the pink colour of the Heart Chakra, via the colour of the petals. There are also two green oils connected with the Heart Chakra, Bergamot and the less well-known Inula. Bergamot opens the Heart Chakra and helps the love-energy to radiate out. Inula is a delicate pale green, but far from delicate in its action and character! It brings moral courage and assists those who are afraid to acknowledge their own highest gifts and exercise them to the full. Melissa, though not green, has a 'green' aroma, and we can relate this oil to the Heart Chakra because of its deeply healing properties at times of grief and separation.

Inula and Melissa can also be valuable where there is some blockage of energy between the Solar Plexus and the Heart, which is not at all unusual. Use one of these oils on the area in between these two chakras to release blocks.

Jasmine warms the Heart Chakra and, through its connection to both the Sacral and Brow Chakras, helps the Heart's function as the point of balance between upper and lower chakras.

The Throat Chakra

Two or three oils are particularly appropriate for the centre of expression. Blue (German) Camomile has always been associated with the Throat Chakra (the colour link is obvious here). It imparts calm strength and enables the truth to be spoken without anger. English Camomile (Anthemis nobilis) is a very delicate pale blue, and resonates with the Throat Chakra at a very high octave, encouraging the expression of spiritual truths. Occasionally we may go to the other end of the spectrum and use the energising action of Myrrh to help somebody who keeps quiet through fear or lack of confidence.

The Brow Chakra

Here we are concerned with the mind and thought and the cephalic oil Rosemary is important, as you would expect. Used with appropriate visualization or intent, Rosemary connects with the higher levels of mind and brings clarity to our understanding of spiritual truths. Juniper, whose berries correspond to the Brow Chakra colour, indigo, assists clairvoyance – but only when it is applied for altruistic ends. Helichrysum activates the right side of the brain, deepening intuition and facilitating access to the unconscious while Thyme has the opposite effect, stimulating the left brain and all conscious and intellectual effort.

The Crown Chakra

There are quite a number of oils that resonate with the expansive and radiant energy of the Thousand Petalled Lotus. You will see that several of them have affinities with other chakras, too, which reflects the fact that the vibrations of every chakra are united at the Crown. So, as you have already seen, both Jasmine and Rose are connected to Sacral, Heart and Crown chakras symbolizing the spiritual dimension of sexuality. Sandalwood bridges Heaven and Earth in the same way. The higher vibrations of Lavender resonate within the Crown Chakra and this is accentuated if you can obtain Alpine Lavender. Frankincense has long been known as a Crown Chakra oil because of its ability to connect us with the Divine within and without. Rosewood has a very special significance, as it facilitates the opening of the Crown Chakra, allowing the outpouring of radiant light and equally the acceptance of Divine light into the Self. You will remember that this is also a Base Chakra oil, as is Frankincense. These links between the Crown and Base Chakras are highly significant, reminding us that chakra energy forms a circuit, and symbolizing the fact that spirit and matter are not separate, but part of a greater Whole. Perhaps oil of Elemi, whose name means 'As above, so below' best embodies this teaching.

The Eighth and Higher Chakras

One or two oils resonate with the Crown and the Eighth Chakra, in particular Frankincense which connects us with the Divine, both within ourselves and without. Lavender, too, resonates with the very high spiritual energy of the Eighth and Ninth Chakras, but the oil which has the strongest connection with these spiritual centres is Neroli. The energy of Neroli is pure, cool and transparent, and encourages our highest aspirations.

Oils for the Lesser Chakras

When working with people who are ungrounded, it is beneficial to include the chakras in the feet, as well as the Base Chakra. The grounding oils described in connection with the Base Chakra are useful here, with Patchouli and Vetivert being the most appropriate.

The chakras at the knees are often blocked or depleted in people who are uncertain or hesitant about their path in life, and those who know in which direction they wish to move but feel temporarily blocked. Inula will help the timid or unsure – as you know it has this action at the Heart Chakra, too. When we know in our heart what we should be doing but are fearful about doing it, Inula applied to both Heart and knee chakras can break down the barriers. Myrrh is another oil that helps at this level, and this one is perhaps more applicable for people who feel blocked or stuck.

Rose and Lavender open and activate the chakras in the palms of the hands and applying one drop of Lavender to each palm before giving healing or massage increases sensitivity to another person's vibrations. Rose links the hands to the Heart and channels love energy from the heart via the hands.

These, then, are the oils to which I feel most strongly drawn when engaging in chakra work, but they do not by any means constitute an exhaustive or exclusive list. I may use other oils at times, according to individual needs and the choice may also change according to different samples of oil. As you know, essential oils vary from season to season and depending on the methods of cultivation, the country of origin and other factors, and even these slight variations can change the subtle energy. To take just one example, I have some Palmarosa oil from Nepal which I would unhesitatingly use for Heart Chakra work, but I do not list Palmarosa as a Heart Chakra oil because most Palmarosa is quite unsuitable. Experiment with an open mind and great sensitivity, using your intuition. The best way to find out how oils relate to chakras is to use them yourself. You do not even need to put them on your body – just inhaling an oil while visualizing a specific chakra will influence the energy. The chakra-diagnosis system outlined below is a very simple way of determining the 'before and after' states of energy and will help you see what effect each oil has when you use it, but try also to feel this within yourself.

When working with chakra energy, essential oils and crystals form a particularly harmonious and beneficial partnership, and this will be explored in the following chapter.

If you are new to chakra work it can be very useful to have a way of investigating the state of each chakra at a specific time, though if you are already accustomed to feeling subtle changes in energy through auric massage or similar work, you will probably find it quite easy to sense what is happening in the various chakras. All the same, the following system of chakra diagnosis using a pendulum can be very valuable. Even therapists who have been working with chakra energy for a long time find it helpful to use this system for a number of reasons.

First, and most important, it allows the therapist to 'see' what is happening in all or any chakra without putting hands, crystals or a pendulum on or near the body. When you bring your hands within another person's aura, especially in the vicinity of any chakra, some change in the energy state is bound to take place, even though it may be slight. If you use a pendulum directly over the body for chakra diagnosis, this can radically alter what is happening at the vibrational level. Dowsing to find the energy state avoids influencing the chakras in any way.

Second, you can dowse for a person who is not physically present, provided you have something, such as a handwriting sample, that makes a link with the person.

Third, you can use this technique for self-diagnosis.

Fourth, by repeating the dowsing after aromatherapy or other appropriate work, you can see immediately what changes have taken place. You can also show this to the person concerned so that they can see this quite graphically for themselves.

Finally, it provides you with a visible record on paper that can be filed and referred to at a later date. This is invaluable if you wish to trace changing energetic patterns over a period of time.

The technique is very simple. Draw the outline of a human body (a stick-person will do perfectly well) and mark on it a dot at the location of each of the major chakras. It is even better if the person for whom you are going to dowse does this personally.

If you use this technique often you would probably find it convenient to have photocopies of a simple outline drawing, in which case ask the person you are working with to draw in the dots. The only basic requirement is that the drawing is big enough to allow space between each chakra for the pendulum to swing clearly over each one.

Hold the pendulum over the dot representing the Base Chakra and watch carefully as it swings. While you are doing this, keep your free hand in contact with the person for whom you are dowsing. If you are doing it for somebody absent, you should try to hold a picture of that person in your mind.

Now mark on the diagram the shape, size and direction of your pendulum's movement. It is best if you do this with a coloured pencil, felt-tip, etc. corresponding to the chakra colour. At this stage, don't try to analyze the pendulum's swing or what it signifies – just record it. Draw a circle, ellipse or line, depending on how the pendulum reacts, and put in some little arrows to show the direction of the swing. If it doesn't move at all, just make a dot in the appropriate colour. The significance of the shapes and sizes will be clearer when you have completed the whole diagram.

Repeat this for each chakra in turn, using the appropriate colour for each one if possible. If you want to include the Eighth or higher chakras, you might like to use the gold or silver metallic-ink pens stocked by many stationers.

Now you can start interpreting your picture. The different shapes that the pendulum may trace each signify a different state of energy.

A circle shows a chakra in good 'health' and functioning as it should. Larger or smaller circles indicate a greater or lesser amount of energy present.

An ellipse suggests that the chakra is in the process of closing. This may be because the individual has decided to close that chakra, in which case the top of the ellipse will be leaning to the right, or it may be that the chakra is closing involuntarily, in which case the ellipse will lean towards the left.

A straight line indicates a closed or almost-closed chakra,

and will point to the right or left in the same way as an ellipse.

If you have made a dot because the pendulum did not move at all, the chakra is in a state of confusion.

When all the chakras are perfectly balanced, both in themselves and in the way they relate to each other, the final diagram will show a series of circles more or less the same size. The direction of swing shown by the arrows will, ideally, alternate with one going clockwise, the next anti-clockwise and so forth.

Once you have your complete diagram in front of you, it will help you decide what is needed to bring all the chakras into better balance. You may need to strengthen the energy in some chakras and pacify others, or encourage more movement of energy between one chakra and another. If there is a very noticeable difference between the size and shape for one chakra on your diagram and the one immediately above or below it, there is some block preventing energy moving freely between them. If you see a marked difference between the state of the three upper chakras and the three lower ones, energy is not moving freely at the Heart Chakra which, you will remember, is the link between the upper and lower centres.

Figure 5 shows this very clearly. This is the chart of a real though, of course, anonymous client. You can see on her chart that all the lower chakras are closed. The Sacral Chakra relating to sex and creativity has been closed down intentionally. The Heart Chakra, though open, lacks a great deal of energy. While the Throat shows a strong, open energy, the Brow Chakra is almost non-functioning, and the Crown Chakra is very big in relation to the others. A pattern similar to this suggests that the lower centres are not being fed by the energy that is certainly present in the upper ones.

The life-situation of this person relates very closely to what the diagram suggests. At the time of this dowsing, she

113

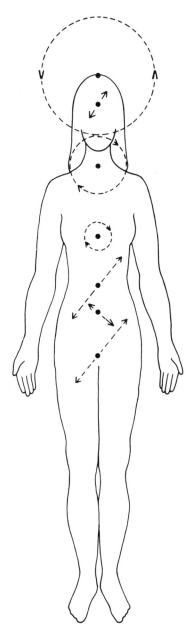

Figure 5

had been divorced for several years, and had been badly hurt in a new relationship that she had entered very soon after the marriage breakdown. She was working in a routine and boring job that allowed no scope for her intellectual or creative capacities. She had embarked some years previously on a programme of meditation and religious studies which gave her great comfort. When I discussed the chart with her, she was very amused by the Sacral and Brow Chakra diagrams, agreeing that she had deliberately shut herself off from any idea of another sexual relationship in the near future and that her job made her feel brain-dead!

Figure 6 shows the same woman's energy pattern after a healing session using essential oils and crystals. You can see straight away that there is far greater balance. Even though the Crown Chakra energy still extends much further than any of the others, this is in accordance with her own desire for spiritual growth and demonstrates how her meditation practice has developed this Chakra.

Of course, to achieve a lasting balance this woman needed some life changes as well as chakra-balance work, but these did follow in due course. The value of chakra balancing is that it facilitates change. When the inner vibrational state changes it allows outer change to happen.

Working with essential oils, crystals or both together (which will be explored in the next chapter) are not the only ways of changing chakra energy. Chanting, visualization and meditation all alter chakra energy, generally bringing about increased energy and better balance. So do expressive activities such as dancing, singing, free drawing or painting or even going into the middle of a field and yelling! Yoga is, of course, supremely balancing and more vigorous forms of exercise are helpful, especially if the lower chakras look depleted or blocked by comparison with the upper ones. The woman described above could have benefited from more exercise, as Figure 6 suggests.

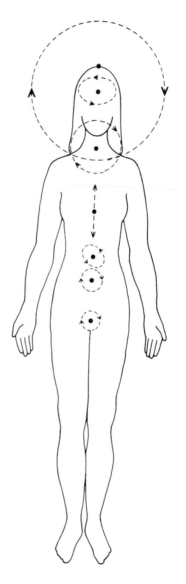

Figure 6

You might want to suggest some of these possibilities if your clients or friends could benefit from them, and of course, as a healer you need to look after the flow and balance of your own energies.

Here is a chakra visualization which you might like to do yourself or suggest to your clients. Before starting this exercise, either put some Vetivert in a burner, or a drop on a tissue to inhale.

Sitting in any comfortable position, focus your attention on the area of the Base Chakra, and imagine a beautiful red flower in bud at the centre of the chakra. Watch the petals unfold. As the flower reaches its fullest size, glowing red light radiates outwards from it, expanding to fill every part of your body. Feel the cells of your body permeated by the red light, and then the whole of your auric field, as the red glow grows and extends far beyond the limits of your physical body. Bring your awareness next to the Sacral Chakra, and see there an orange-coloured flower in bud, which radiates an ever-expanding light in the same way as before.

Repeat this for each of the chakras in turn, seeing at each one a flower of the appropriate colour. Try to experience the feeling of each different colour, not merely look at it. What does your body feel like when it is filled with red? with blue? and so on.

When you have moved through each of the chakras in this way, it is important to close them again. To be too open can leave you vulnerable to some outside energies you might prefer not to invite into your very personal space.

Do this in the reverse order, beginning with the Crown Chakra, where we watch the flower move from a full bloom to a bud, from a bud to a tiny point of light. Then, in your imagination, draw circle anticlockwise where the flower has been, and a cross within the circle.

Repeat this with each of the chakras in order, ending with the Base.

It is also important to close the chakras before going into crowded places, before meeting people you find difficult or any situation that makes you feel threatened. Equally, you should close or protect yourself before working with clients, to avoid depletion of your own energy. You may well already have a way of doing this that feels appropriate, but if you do not, the second half of this visualization is an effective protection. Once you are accustomed to it, you will find that you can do it really quickly whenever you need to.

CHAPTER 9

Crystals and Oils – A Healing Partnership

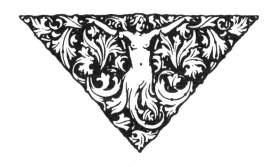

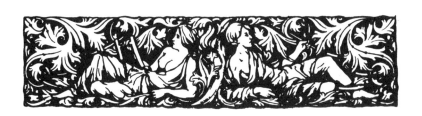

Crystals are powerful allies of the subtle healer in their own right, as are essential oils, of course, but by bringing the two together in harmony we can enhance their healing power still further.

This can be done in a number of ways, from simply having healing crystals nearby while carrying out conventional aromatherapy treatments right through to vaporising essential oil in the room when giving crystal healing.

Before considering some of the possibilities that lie between these two extremes, I will outline, very briefly, the nature of crystals and how they are used in healing. If you find yourself drawn to crystals as healing tools there are some excellent books that can guide you further along that path. Better still, find a teacher in whom you have confidence to teach you at first hand.

Crystals are the most evolved manifestation of the mineral kingdom, standing at a point between organic and inorganic creation. Some scientists think that crystals may hold the secret of the origin of organic life, for they have certain characteristics of living things: they are self-organizing, they can reproduce themselves (by means of seed crystals), they carry information and they receive, hold, amplify and transmit energy. They are able to do so because of their highly-organised structure. This fact is made use of in many scientific and industrial applications, and is equally true in healing. Crystals can channel more life-force into the physical and subtle bodies and channel out negative energies. The frequency of vibration, the speed of transmission and the degree of amplification will depend on many factors, including the size, shape and colour of the crystal, the manner in which it is handled by the healer and the intention of the healer at the time of using the crystal. Indeed, to say that crystals magnify and transmit the healer's intent could be a summary of crystal healing. Different healers use their crystals in different ways, but the underlying principles remain the same.

Crystals can be divided into two categories: colourless/transparent crystals such as quartz, and coloured crystals or gemstones, and the two groups are used in different ways for healing. The most widely used healing crystals are quartz which may be completely transparent, smoky (grey) or slightly milky in appearance. Some healers describe the completely clear crystals as masculine and the milky ones as feminine but this is by no means a hard and fast rule. Indeed, nothing connected with crystals should be considered as a fixed rule, and I am always wary of teachers who declare that such-and-such a crystal does this (and only this) while such-and-such another crystal does only that. Intuition and an open mind are far more likely to lead you to the right choice of crystal for you and your purpose at any particular moment.

Instead of masculine and feminine, you may find it more helpful to think in terms of giving out and taking in. Most people working with healing energies find that their right hand tends mostly to give out energy, while their left hand detects and identifies or takes in energy, and this is as likely to be true of left-handed people as of right-handed. If you are not sure whether this is true for you, try one of the exercises described in The Role of the Healer. Many crystal healers work with a pair of quartz crystals – one attuned to each hand. The best way to establish whether a particular crystal will work best for you as a transmitter or a receiver is simply to hold it in your hands and respond sensitively to the way it feels. Take the crystal in your right hand and bring it close to your solar plexus, holding it for a few minutes, then transfer it to your left hand until you get a feeling of where it seems most comfortable to you. Then bring the crystal close to your heart and welcome it. Finally, give thanks for this gift from the earth that will help you in your healing work. Do this whenever you buy or are given a new crystal.

The coloured crystals or gemstones are used somewhat differently, and their colour is usually the factor that indicates their use because it suggests what the vibration of that stone is like. Clear quartz crystals, by reason of their transparency and absence of colour, can resonate with any frequency of vibrations. The coloured stones, on the other hand are each attuned to a narrower range of vibrations that correspond to their colour. They are often used to influence chakra energy and chosen for their correspondence to the colours associated with each chakra: dark reddish, brown or black stones with the Base Chakra, orange with the Sacral and so on. However, the choice will also depend on what kind of energy input is needed at that chakra. If you feel there is a need to stimulate, a red stone may be the most appropriate regardless of which chakra you are dealing with, while green or pale blue crystals can be used to calm, soothe or cool.

Many of the coloured crystals can be related to essential oils that have similar actions, and quite often you will find that there is a correspondence in colour. Sometimes this will be very obvious, as when the crystal and the essential oil itself are the same colour but at times you may need to look further than the oil and seek a correlation between the colour of the stone and that of the flower, etc. from which the oil was obtained.

To take an example: Rose quartz harmonizes exquisitely with Rose absolute. Both relate to the Heart Chakra and to love of many kinds from the romantic and sexual to the love of a mother for her child. Here we can see a relationship between the colour of the crystal and that of the parent flower, as we can when we compare the healing properties of Lavender with those of amethyst. Blue Camomile oil, on the other hand, has a more obvious connection with such blue stones as lapis, blue lace agate, etc., which share its ability to calm and soothe.

Sometimes the connection is harder to understand, and may have more to do with the actual aroma of the oil than its appearance, or the appearance of its parent plant. It may help to bear in mind that such terms as 'green', 'fresh', 'dark', 'heavy' and so forth are often used to describe aromas, so an oil with a green scent might be found to have an affinity for a green gemstone, etc. To take an example once again, Sandalwood, though light in colour has a dark aroma, and can be likened in many ways to the gemstone known as Tiger's Eye, which is brown streaked with gold.

There are many essential oils and crystals which resonate with each other in terms of their vibrations and their healing action and which have the same colour, either literally or less obviously, but do not be too rigid in applying this principle to the harmonising of an oil to a crystal. If you do, you might miss some wonderful revelations! What is important is that the vibration, or energy-quality of the oil and the crystal are in harmony with each other: the colour of each is often an indication of the vibrational energy, rather than a factor that is important in its own right.

In each of our examples the oil and the crystal could be said to resonate together: in other words, they work in harmony with each other and we can reasonably assume that in terms of healing energy they produce a similar vibration. Certainly in terms of observable effect, such combinations are sometimes almost miraculously potent.

To return for a moment to the clear crystals: because they are in themselves without colour, they are able to resonate with every colour in the spectrum, so you may use quartz crystals with any essential oil.

One of the simplest ways to use crystals in conjunction with aromatherapy, especially if subtle aromatherapy is a relatively new field for you, is to place a small crystal in your dish of massage oil to potentise it. If you do, please remember to use the lowest percentage of essential oil in the mixture: 1%, or even as little as a half percent if you are using a highly-perfumed oil. Crystal energy is very powerful in its own right, and the standard amounts of essential oil would be quite overpowering when the two forms of healing energy are brought together.

Another simple way of combining the two energies is to place a crystal at each corner of the massage table while you are working (Figure 7). For this you can use two pairs of quartz crystals which should ideally be fairly evenly matched in size, or you can use coloured crystals if these are appropriate to your client's needs. If you are new to working with crystals, you may not have a large number to work with, in which case the choice may depend on what crystals you have available to use, and what you hope to achieve. Whichever you choose, the aim should be to enhance the action of the essential oil or blend you are using.

For example, if you are working with somebody who feels very depleted and lacking in energy you could place all four crystals with their points facing inwards towards the body in order to channel more energy in, but if you are dealing with somebody who is over-stimulated, restless, excitable, unable to sleep, etc., you might place your four crystals pointing outwards to draw off some of the excess energy. The same arrangement of crystals can be used to draw out negative energy, for example, if your client has been in a crowded place, public transport, etc. Do remember, though, that whenever energy is taken out, something must take its place, so you would need to finish the healing session by channelling in some pure, healing energy, either by turning the crystals around, or with a crystal wand if you have one or through your choice of essential oil.

An alternative scheme is to have a single crystal just above the crown of the person's head, and two at the feet as before

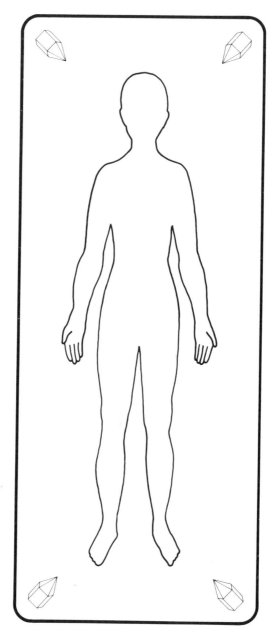

Figure 7

(Figure 8). Whichever configuration you use, visualise white light running between the crystals to form a circle of light round the person with whom you are working.

It is not difficult to see how the placing of your crystals correlates with your choice of oils. In the examples I have given, you could place the crystals pointing inwards to increase energy while using tonic or stimulating oils such as Rosemary, Thyme, etc. In the second example, you might want soothing or sedative oils such as Lavender, Bergamot, etc., or perhaps a detoxifying oil like Juniper. But remember that crystals work with your intent and will increase the potency of whatever oils you use, so you will need to make lower dilutions than you would normally use. If you are doing direct bodywork, aimed at alleviating a physical problem, you could use up to 2% dilution but if you are engaged in more subtle, energetic work you would need to use a very low dilution indeed: perhaps as little as a half percent.

If you think that the crystals will impede your movements while massaging, simply place them on the floor underneath the couch, directly below the four corners. (Do remember, though, to take care of your crystals by placing each one on a cloth, preferably silk, or on top of its own carrying pouch.)

Another crystal that can beneficially be placed under a massage couch is amethyst. Amethysts absorb and transmute negative energies, so they can help both the giver and the receiver in a healing session. The best form of amethyst to use for this purpose is a cluster. You might place one on the floor under the massage couch or at the bottom of the couch between your client's feet and 'ask' it to transmute any negative energy released during the session. If you have clients who you think might be sceptical about the use of crystals in this way, you might simply place an amethyst cluster on a shelf or windowsill where – if they notice it at all – it can pass for an item of decoration! Your more

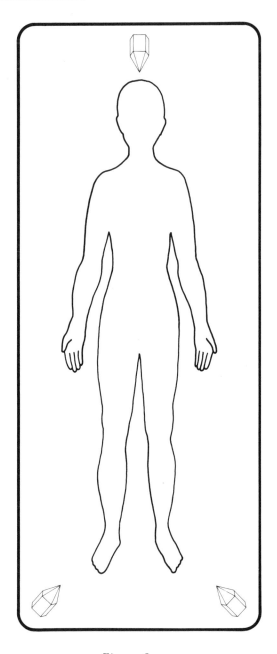

Figure 8

sensitive clients will appreciate your crystals for their true worth and the more you practise subtle aromatherapy the more likely you are to attract clients who wish to work with you at a subtle level.

Rose quartz is another crystal that enhances all forms of aromatherapy. It evokes love and healing at very deep levels. It has a very special affinity with the Heart Chakra, so I often place a rose quartz below the couch directly under the client's heart centre.

You might like to use a crystal to carry out auric massage. If you have an egg-shaped crystal or a small sphere you can very gently massage the aura with that, or you can use one of the long sides of a straight crystal. A single drop of essential oil can be placed on the crystal before you begin work.

Very tiny, finely pointed crystals are sometimes used to apply energy to an acupuncture or shiatsu point on the physical body, or to corresponding points within the aura and here again you can put a drop of an appropriate oil on your crystal. Such small crystals are usually set in a metal wand which makes them easier to hold and to use with precision.

Even when using traditional aromatherapy, you will often find that your client feels a little light-headed or detached from the 'real' world at the end of a massage, and this is often more noticeable when you have been working with the aura, the Chakras or in other subtle ways. To counteract this, you can place at the foot end of the couch one or more crystals that have a grounding and earthing effect. Place a single, biggish, crystal centrally on the couch between your client's feet, or a smaller stone just below each foot. Any dark-coloured gemstone is suitable, but a particularly good choice would be Hematite. Hematite is very dense (it is a form of iron ore) and very grounding. You will usually find this stone in small rounded pieces or egg shapes polished to a dark silver. In its original state, before polishing, hematite is a deep brownish-red resembling a kidney and when split open its surface patterning is also kidney-like. You could say that hematite acts in relation to the subtle bodies in the same way that our kidneys act in relation to our physical bodies: absorbing toxins and flushing them away so if you feel that anybody has a lot of 'psychic junk' that needs to be channelled away, give them a hematite to hold in each hand.

Another crystal that effectively absorbs negative energy of all kinds is smoky quartz.

Crystals also enhance essential oils by amplifying the aroma. Just one drop of oil on a crystal will perfume an entire room. Putting oils on crystals also makes the aroma last longer, sometimes for several days, even with the most fugitive perfumes.

Crystals and essential oils can be combined for the purpose of absent healing. If you have sufficient information about the person who needs healing to select an appropriate oil for that person's needs, it is good to do so. Or meditate silently for a few minutes and ask for guidance, or use your intuitive insight to choose the right oil. Put a single drop of oil on a suitable crystal and place the crystal in front of you while you visualize the person in perfect health, or send healing in whatever way you are accustomed to do. Use the largest crystal you can, but do not worry if you do not have a very big quartz crystal: use whatever you have and remember that your intent is what is important. A genuine, altruistic desire to promote healing is more important than the particular crystal you use.

If you meet in a group for absent healing, place the crystal with its drop of oil in the centre of your circle. Healing groups most often work for a number of individuals at each of their sessions, so a generally healing oil with wide-ranging properties, such as Lavender, is probably the most appropriate to use. Bach Flower Remedies, other Flower

Essences, Gem Elixirs and homeopathic remedies can be placed on a crystal for absent healing in exactly the same way.

So far, we have mostly considered ways in which crystals enhance essential oils, but the converse is also true. The oils can be used to energise crystals and to clean them. If you have a crystal that looks a little dull and lifeless, try putting a drop of essential oil on it and see what happens. Choose an oil that you think is attuned to that crystal.

Essential oils can be used to clean crystals as an alternative to the more usual methods of cleaning with salt water or purifying smoke. A crystal will need cleaning every time it has been used in healing. Crystals that are worn on the body, such as crystal pendants, etc., need cleaning once a week, and crystals that are kept in rooms need cleaning at least once a month – more often if the space is used for healing work, or if any negativity is felt: for example if there has been an angry confrontation in the room.

When I am at home I clean my crystals in the traditional way with salt water. For this, take some sea-salt and dissolve it in natural spring water so that the water is saturated (i.e. it will not hold any more salt). Leave clear crystals in this overnight to cleanse. It is important to use natural sea-salt and spring water, not tapwater, for this because sea-salt and spring water have a coherent structure, resembling that of crystals (indeed, sea-salt is crystal). Crystals that have been mounted in silver to wear as a pendant or other form of jewellery should not be left overnight in salt water, nor should the coloured gemstones. Instead wipe them with spring water on a silk or cotton cloth (no synthetics) and, if possible, place them in the sunlight.

All crystals benefit from being put in sunlight whenever possible. In summer, I sometimes put my whole collection out in the garden to sunbathe. If a crystal has been used for very deep healing work such as with people who are terminally ill, the crystal may need to be rested for quite a long time and then you should bury it in the earth for a month or more. Remember that all crystals are the Earth's gift to us so resting in the earth is like going home.

Another method of cleansing is to smoke or 'smudge' the crystals. This the way traditionally used by native American Indians, holding the crystals in the smoke of the traditional smudging herbs Cedar, Sage and Sweetgrass. An alternative is to bury the crystals for a week or longer in a bowl of cleansing herbs, such as Cedar, Juniper, Lavender, Mugwort, Pine, Rosemary, Rosewood or Sage (Salvia).

As you will realise immediately, every one of these herbs yields an essential oil, so you could perfectly well cleanse your crystals with one or more of the oils instead. Put three to four drops of oil in an essential oil burner, and hold your crystal or crystals in the vapour when it begins to rise. I sometimes add a drop of Lemongrass to take the place of Sweetgrass which is not obtainable in the form of essential oil. Neither the 'Sage' nor the 'Cedar' in authentic smudge sticks are the same species that we use in aromatherapy, but their ability to cleanse are the same, so the substitution is quite valid.

Essential oils are specially useful for cleaning crystals if you are not in your own home, or healing centre, because you need no equipment. Simply take a drop of oil and wipe the crystal with it. If you have a cotton cloth, such as a clean hankie, put the oil on that but I have used tissues for this purpose when nothing else was available.

Having looked at ways in which crystals can enhance essential oils and vice versa, I now come to the important area of Chakra balancing and healing, where the two act together in a healing harmony. In the preceding chapter we looked at how various essential oils related to different chakras, and how they could be used to heal and balance chakra energy. Now that we have explored together a small corner of the vast world of crystals, we can bring these two areas of knowledge together and see how they meet, overlap and potentise each other.

Before I outline some of the crystals and essential oils that harmonize with each other, and the chakras to which they relate, I would like to explain how these associations were arrived at. For some years I had been using crystals in aromatherapy treatments in the simple ways suggested above, and was wishing to expand and deepen my knowledge of crystals when I came across two teachers who I instinctively felt were the people from whom I wanted to learn. About a year after I completed their course, and had been working in various ways with crystals, they mentioned to me that they had long wanted to do more work combining crystals with essential oils, and asked if I would like to do some joint work with them. Thus began an exciting exploration, some of the results of which are set out below.

As the relationship between the various essential oils and the chakras has been discussed fairly fully in the previous chapter, I will do little more than mention the relevant oils unless more detail is needed to explain how or why they harmonise with the different crystals.

The Base Chakra

The black, dark brown and reddish crystals that resonate with the Base Chakra have similar energy-qualities to the Base Chakra oils: grounding, balancing and energizing. In particular, Black Obsidian has a virtually identical vibration to Patchouli, while Hematite resonates with Myrrh. Myrrh is also strongly related to Garnet and other red stones. Black Tourmaline grounds and protects and can be used on the Base, Sacral and Solar Plexus Chakras in harmony with

Vetivert. Frankincense relates to both the Base and the Crown Chakras, and in this it mirrors the stone known as Tiger's Eye which is a brown stone with golden bands. Rosewood is another oil which is applicable to both Base and Crown Chakras, and it is associated with a type of crystal known as Black Tourmalinated Quartz (clear Quartz containing within it bands of Black Tourmaline) which in the same way symbolizes the connection of Crown and Base.

The Sacral Chakra

Crystals and gemstones that affect the Sacral Chakra are often orange or orange-red in colour. The denser (opaque) stones have a quite direct, physical effect on this chakra, while those that resonate at a more subtle level are usually transparent. Citrine has a close affinity with Sandalwood, both at the Sacral Chakra and, in its higher vibrations at the Crown. Rose oil is so rich and diverse in its vibrations that it relates to a number of different gemstones. At the Sacral Chakra, Rose relates most strongly with Ruby, which gives warmth and strength. Jasmine, equally rich and varied, resonates in total harmony with Sapphire, at every level – Sacral, Heart and Crown Chakras. This may come as a surprise, as it breaks with virtually all expectations, but in fact the correspondence between this oil and stone is total. Jasmine also works harmoniously at Sacral level with Red Jasper and with the warming, stimulating effects of Ruby.

The Solar Plexus Chakra

Juniper, which as you know, is a cleanser, especially for the Solar Plexus, finds a perfect partner in Sulphur which is equally cleansing in its action. Vetivert may be used in tandem with Yellow Jasper or the Black Tourmaline with which it is equally active at the Base, Sacral and Solar Plexus centres.

The Heart Chakra

Rose, as mentioned in relation to the Sacral Chakra is so complex that no single stone exactly corresponds to it at all levels. Rose Quartz certainly harmonises with the warm, loving energy of Rose at Earth level (but only if it is gem quality). Rose goes beyond that, though, and we find an affinity with Ruby at the Heart Level as well as the Sacral. At a higher, more spiritual and universal level Rose resonates more with Kunzite, Just as Rose oil is so beautifully attuned to babies and children, Kunzite is a stone for children, to help keep their souls intact. Kunzite expands Heart energy upwards, whereas Watermelon Tourmaline expands outwards and has very much the same kind of energy as Bergamot. Watermelon Tourmaline is a delicately tinted stone, pink in the centre surrounded by pale green, thereby matching completely the pink/green energy of the Heart Centre.

Inula, the other green oil associated with the Heart Chakra resonates with the light green stone, Aventurine to a degree that is almost uncanny: Aventurine's properties being identical with those of the oil.

Malachite is another green stone, which is associated not so much with the Heart Chakra as with the movement of energy between the Solar Plexus and Heart. Blocks which prevent energy moving as it should from Solar Plexus to Heart level are often the result of a past event, maybe buried deep, and Malachite can bring things up from a very deep level. No less than three essential oils work in harmony with this stone: Black Pepper, Carrotseed and Sage. Black Pepper is a 'shifter' as is Malachite. Malachite is also associated with inner sight, and carrots have long been reputed to improve the eyesight: at a symbolic level both the oil and the stone help the user to 'see in the dark'. Lastly, Malachite cleanses, it is an emotional purger, and thus relates to the third of its companion oils, Sage, which is likewise a purging and purifying herb. Before working with Malachite, with or without essential oils, you should be aware that although it does bring past events and emotions to the surface, it does not get rid of them, so some other means is needed to do that – either different oils and stones, or perhaps counselling or therapy work. Working with Malachite can be confrontational and you should ask anybody for whom you might use this stone whether they are willing.

The Throat Chakra

At the Throat Chakra we again find a clear colour correspondence, with Blue Camomile having an energy-quality very close to that of Blue Tourmaline. This is the dark blue German Camomile, but there is an equal degree of harmony when we look at the higher vibrations of the Throat Chakra, where the pale blue English Camomile resonates with three light blue stones, Aquamarine, Amazonite and Aqua Aura. All these are concerned with the higher purpose of the Throat Chakra, in expressing spiritual truth. Comparison between Camomile and Aqua Aura is particularly fascinating. This is not a naturally-occurring stone, but is made by placing clear Quartz in a closed chamber with gold atoms and subjecting it to high temperatures. Camomile oils, obtained from the little white and gold flowers by distillation at high temperature, are not naturally blue – the coloration only appears during the distillation process.

The Brow Chakra

Oils that connect with the Brow Chakra also have some clear correspondences with gemstones. Here, the affinity is not indicated very clearly by colour, but the actions of the twinned stones and oils are virtually identical. Rosemary resonates with Sujalite, both being concerned with clear vision and clairvoyance. Thyme, connecting with the conscious, intellectual mind, parallels the energy of Sodalite, and the qualities of Helichrysum link it to two stones, Kyanite and Lapis Lazuli. Lapis, in particular, opens up compassion.

The Crown Chakra

A whole constellation of stones and oils cluster at the Thousand Petalled Lotus, reflecting the many different energies that converge and combine here. Several of them have been mentioned before, as they relate to more than one chakra. Rose oil at the Crown Chakra level echoes the delicate vibrations of Pink Calcite and Watermelon Tourmaline, Sandalwood resonates with Citrine at the Crown as well as at the Sacral Chakra. Similarly Jasmine reflects Sapphire energy. The relationship between Frankincense and Tiger's Eye reflects the connection between the Crown Chakra and the Base, the brown stone being of a Base Chakra colour and resonance, while the golden bands within it belong to the golden light radiating from the Crown Chakra. Rosewood at this high level harmonizes with rutilated Smoky Quartz and with Apophylite. Apophylite, a very delicate pale green crystal, expresses the higher level of Heart energy, and we might connect this with love for the Amazon and for our Planet.

Then we find some oils and stones that harmonize only with the Crown Chakra. The pure healing energy of Amethyst is of the same quality as that of Lavender. Mandarin oil, warm but delicate harmonizes with both Pink and Gold Topaz, embodying Christ Child energy.

The vibrations of Elemi are the same in quality as those of Elestials (Skeleton Quartz). This stone stabilises brain waves and neutralizes negative thoughts. It also activates the Crown Chakra, so we might connect it with Rosewood, too,

137

but it can also bring up deeply buried emotions, and has very profound effects. As with Malachite, you should not work with this stone unless the person concerned is willing.

The Eighth and Higher Chakras

The Eighth Chakra is the centre of the higher self, where we reach out towards the Divine. Its energy is pure and expansive, and only one oil fully harmonizes with its purity and radiance. This is Neroli, representing Sun energy in a very refined form. The orange blossom with its pure white petals and golden stamens finds an echo in Herkemer Diamonds which are also white with gold. Fluorite, Rutilated Quartz and even Diamonds match the vibrations of Neroli, but the greatest harmony exists between Neroli and Selenite, a white crystal of the greatest purity and refinement.

Angelica, like Rosewood, is associated with Apophylite and these three may also find expression in the Eighth Chakra, particularly in lifting Crown Chakra energy to this even higher level. Angelica also has affinities with Green Tourmaline, both of them expressing urgent, upward expansion. But Angelica can be likened, too, to Moss Agate or Bloodstone, which has 'root' energy and an earthing effect. Thus we can see that stones, oils and chakra energies come full circle.

Choosing, buying and taking care of crystals must be done just as carefully as selecting and storing essential oils. Quality is every bit as important and in buying crystals you should seek out gem quality stones whenever you can as these have the highest healing vibrations. In certain applications the lower-grade stones are useless because their vibrations are quite different. As with oils, try to buy crystals from suppliers who specialise in stones for healing, rather than decorative or industrial use. They will be knowledgeable about crystals for healing work and they will take care to buy from sources that do not deplete the Earth. Where possible, buy stones that have been hand mined, rather than cut out of the Earth with machines.

When you work with crystals and essential oils together, you should never regard the crystals as merely an adjunct to aromatherapy. They are radiant, beautiful and powerful in their own right. They have their own Devas just as the healing plants and oils do, and when we bring certain aspects of the mineral and the plant kingdoms together it is as if we were inviting their Devas to meet and work together for the purpose of healing. That they do work together so harmoniously is something for which we must never forget to give thanks.

As with so much else in this book, I have outlined the methods that I use and find effective. If you already use crystals in ways that differ from these, of course you should continue, though perhaps you will find something in this chapter to add to your existing repertoire.

CHAPTER 10

Essential Oils and Meditation

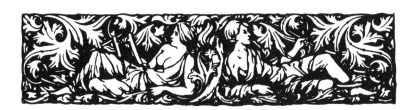

A romatics have been used since time immemorial to facilitate meditation, contemplation and prayer. Incenses and aromatics in one form or another have been an integral part of the practice of virtually every religion, from the shamanistic rituals of primitive man to the great world religions of both East and West. The present century has seen a strong movement towards what we might call secular meditation: meditation that does not form part of a formal religious practice but may be undertaken as a way of promoting personal growth, world peace, the healing of our planet, etc. Aromatics can enhance such practices just as much as meditation in a religious context.

The earliest incenses were simply sprigs of suitable plants, burnt to produce a scented smoke. This method is still used, for example, in the 'smudge stick' used by American Indians to purify places or people. In parts of the world where resin-producing trees are found, people discovered that they could collect the resin and burn it rather than gather, transport and store bulky branches and from the burning of simple resins, the production of complex incenses developed. Some of these resins, such as Frankincense, Myrrh and Elemi are still widely used. Sweetly scented flowers were scattered on altars, or in front of sacred statues, and in India especially, precious perfumes would be poured on the altars, or on the ground near them.

In many cultures, the use of incense or other perfumes was originally intended as an offering to the deity but inhaling these scented smokes also had beneficial effects on the participants. In particular, many traditional incenses have a calming and clarifying effect on the mind, which helps the meditator to set aside mundane thoughts for a while, while others have the physical effect of deepening and slowing the breath, which in itself can help to create a deeply meditative state. How much more do we need such help when we wish to incorporate meditation into busy 20th century lives.

Essential oils can advantageously replace some of the other ways of using aromatics for meditation. They offer us the perfume of the plant in a very pure, very refined form, and make it possible to choose from virtually any aroma, whatever and wherever its origins.

Some of the uses to which essential oils can be put in this context include:

- Purifying and preparing the place where we intend to meditate. If this is in the home, or some place that is not used exclusively for meditation or similar purposes, such preparation may even need to include dispersing cooking, cigarette smoke or other unwanted smells. Using incense or essential oils to perfume a room prior to meditation is a way of dedicating the space and highlights the fact that, for the time being at least, this space is set apart from any mundane use.

- Helping the meditator to set aside day-to-day preoccupations and intrusive thoughts.

- Deepening and slowing the breath. Increasing awareness of the breath and helping the meditator to focus upon it.

- Calming the mind. Increasing mental clarity.

- Balancing chakra energy. Opening the higher chakras.

- Heightening awareness. Raising consciousness to the higher levels.

- Grounding and earthing energy. This may sound contradictory, but can be very important. Extensive meditation practice can leave the meditator feeling very detached from daily life, and unable to function in the physical world. Unless one lives in an enclosed, contemplative community this can be a real handicap. Ideally, meditation should help us to lead better lives at every level, and grounding and earthing aromas can be a real help in this respect.

- Harmonising the energies of individuals in a group. In group meditations each person taking part brings his or her personal energy, thoughts, preoccupations and wishes into the group. When everybody involved inhales the same incense or essential oil this helps to bring the group together as a harmonious whole.

- Finally, we should not lose sight of the original intend of offering aromatics to a deity or higher power. If your personal beliefs include a deity or higher consciousness, it can be very beautiful and meaningful to make an offering of your essential oil. If not, you might wish to dedicate the aromatic offering to world peace, to individual or planetary healing, or to your own higher self, whichever feels most appropriate. When pouring the oil focus your mind on the purpose of the meditation for which you are using it, the benefits which you hope to obtain from it for yourself or others and mentally offer the oil to the highest good.

METHODS OF USE

The most suitable ways to use essential oils as an aid to meditation are in burners and diffusers. Diffusers are not really appropriate for use during an actual meditation, because they make some noise, which can be irritating and distracting. However, they are very good indeed for filling a room quickly with the chosen aroma which makes them suitable for preparing a room beforehand. The larger diffusers designed for clinical or commercial use are excellent if you are going to use a relatively large space.

The more traditional burners are better for using during meditation as they are soundless and they have the added attraction of producing a gentle light at the same time. Both burners and diffusers are useful for either personal or group meditations.

When meditating alone, you could put a drop or two of your chosen oil in a tissue or handkerchief as an alternative, and simply placing this where you can smell it during your meditation. Or you may like to place a single drop of an appropriate oil on one or more chakras before your sitting, perhaps on the Crown Chakra to increase spiritual awareness, or on the Heart Chakra to promote feelings of compassion. Many people like to do this as a preparation and then burn the same or a compatible oil while they are actually sitting.

HELPFUL OILS

A number of oils are helpful for meditation. Many of them are obtained from the same plants and trees that have traditionally been used as incense for thousands of years. You will find a more detailed account of each of these oils in another section, but the following notes should serve as a guide to choosing the most appropriate for your meditations.

ANGELICA Helps us to come into closer contact with the divine.

CEDARWOOD This has been traditionally used as an incense (often with Juniper) in Tibet and Nepal.

FRANKINCENSE One of the most ancient and widely used incenses, Frankincense deepens and slows the rate of breathing. This helps to bring about a calm and meditative state.

ELEMI Less well known, Elemi comes from a tree closely related to frankincense and has similar properties. It has perhaps less impact on the breath, but is more balancing and grounding and some people find that it facilitates visualization.

146

HELICHRYSUM Activates the intuitive side of the brain, which may help with meditations that involve visualization, guided imagery, etc.

JUNIPER Is a psychic cleanser, as well as a physical detoxifier. Very good for clearing rooms before meditation.

LAVENDER Another balancing oil. As it is also sedative, it is best used in a blend with other oils, particularly Rosemary, in order to avoid drowsiness while meditating.

ROSE Opens the Heart Chakra, allowing love to be given and received. Stimulates creativity, which can help in meditations that involve visualization, especially for people who find this kind of work difficult. A very costly oil, this may feel appropriate to dedicate as an offering on very special occasions.

ROSEMARY Is a spiritual protector, so another good oil for clearing rooms that are not normally used for meditation. It promotes mental clarity. Best used in a blend so that its stimulant properties do not offset its other benefits. It may be wise not to use this oil for evening meditation.

CAUTION: Do not use for anybody who suffers from epilepsy or high blood pressure.

ROSEWOOD Has the ability to open the Crown Chakra, if the individual is ready for this to happen. Creates a feeling of calm without inducing drowsiness.

SANDALWOOD Another traditional incense. Very calming. Moderately grounding.

VETIVERT Has a balancing action, very good for bringing the energy of all major chakras into alignment, and for harmonising group energies. Very calming and grounding.

These are the oils most often used as meditational aids, but as you become familiar with the subtle qualities of essential oils you will find that virtually every one of them is able to enhance meditation in some way, and that your choice will intuitively be guided towards the oil that best fits your own needs and the particular meditation you envisage.

CHAPTER 11

Flower Remedies in Subtle Aromatherapy

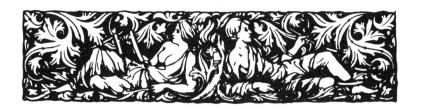

The Flower Remedies or Flower Essences could be described as the most subtle of all forms of plant healing. Unlike essential oils, they contain no measurable material from the original plant, in which they bear more resemblance to homeopathic remedies. Indeed, the originator of Flower Remedies, Dr. Edward Bach, was trained in homeopathy as well as orthodox medicine.

The Remedies are prepared, in most instances, by floating the chosen flowers on a container of pure spring water and placing this in sunlight for several hours. During this time, something of the plant's energy is transferred to the spring water and it is this energy that is the healing factor in the eventual Remedy. Nothing else is added to the energised spring water except a little brandy to act as a preservative.

Flower Remedies act on the mental, emotional and personality levels, though physical healing often takes place as a result of the less obvious effects.

Each of the 38 plants which make up the original repertoire of Flower Remedies was discovered by a highly intuitive process. A highly sensitive person, Dr. Bach would often develop the very symptoms or emotional stresses that a certain plant was destined to relieve, and would then find himself drawn to the appropriate plant.

His discoveries were made during the 1930s and in recent decades the repertoire has been vastly expanded by individuals and groups of people in many parts of the world who are finding new remedies (often known as Flower Essences) among the plants in their own localities. Some of these have been found intuitively, but many of the new Essences have been found as a result of channelled information. This work has been, and is currently, going on in England and Scotland, in Australia, in Alaska, Arizona, California, Virginia and other parts of the U.S.A. (and I apologise to anybody whose work has not yet come to my attention). It is inevitable that new remedies should emerge at the present time, as many of our needs are radically different from those of people living over 50 years ago. That is not to say that Dr. Bach's Remedies are no longer needed, for he addressed many fundamental aspects of the human psyche, but neither he nor his patients were subject to heavy environmental pollution, fear of nuclear annihilation or many of the stresses of late-twentieth-century society. For these, new remedies are needed, and have appeared. For example, we find several remedies to help reduce the stress of urban living.

Another, perhaps more positive, reason why the newer Flower Essences have come into being is that as the world enters the dawn of a New Age, a vast and ever-growing number of individuals seek to attune themselves to the changing planetary energy, to a higher level of being. Such attunement involves much inner work which may encompass prayer, meditation, visualization, affirmation, workshops, individual therapy, past-life regression or what-ever other means are appropriate for the individual. Subtle aromatherapy is a valuable adjunct to such work, and so are the new Flower Essences. Many of them are concerned with the soul's journey, with past-life experiences and the move-ment towards a greater spirituality in every aspect of life. This is particularly true of the Alaskan and Virginian essences. It is in this aspect of our work that the Essences and essential oils so beautifully enhance each other.

On the subject of how to use Flower Essences jointly with Subtle Aromatherapy, there is not, in fact, very much to say. The most usual method is to select a suitable Flower Remedy or Essence to be taken by mouth in the usual way. This may either reinforce the action of the essential oil(s) through a similarity of vibration, or more often complement it by bringing in a different vibration – maybe one that none of your oils embodies.

It is usual to dowse to decide on the Flower Essence or

combination of Essences to use. Even for people who work all the time with Flower Essences and are highly familiar with them, this is probably the best way to choose as it allows the intuition free reign and prevents the practitioner being influenced in any way by what he or she knows about the Essences.

One of the reasons why Flower Essences and essential oils complement each other so well is that, for the most part, they are prepared from different ranges of plants. There are some overlaps, of course, where an essential oil and a Flower Essence are prepared from the same plant, but they are relatively few. This means that a practitioner using essential oils can draw on a Flower Essence to provide a particular vibration that cannot be found in any of the essential oils, and the converse, of course, is just as true. Flower Essences can be prepared from plants that have little or no perfume and would not therefore yield any essential oil, so they greatly enlarge the range of plants with which we can work. Even where an oil and a Flower Essence from the same plant do exist, they will not be identical in their vibrations or their action, but each will enhance the action of the other by working in a slightly different way.

Recently, though, I have met one or two therapists who take this a step further and actually add a drop or two of the chosen Flower Essence to their massage oil. This they do for exactly the same reason: to bring into the blend a vibrational quality that complements that of the essential oil(s). Having been 'on the receiving end' of such treatments several times, I can testify to their profound effect. Another couple are developing Remedies which combine both flower and gem essences, and several groups have been working on environmental essences, i.e. essences which capture the spirit of a time such as the Summer Solstice, or a special and healing place like Lourdes.

Doubtless some of these new methods are unorthodox, whether viewed from the traditional aromatherapist's standpoint or that of the Flower Essence practitioner, but imaginative innovations are part of the development of all areas of subtle therapy and point the way forward for us all.

CHAPTER 12

Sex, Spirit and Essential Oils

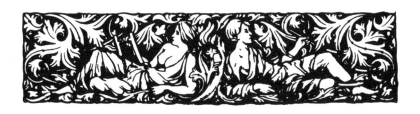

S ome of the essential oils that are used as meditational aids are also renowned aphrodisiacs. This may seem contradictory, for sex and spirituality are so often thought of as antipathetic. Indeed, many spiritual traditions place great emphasis on celibacy, whether in a celibate priesthood or in monastic and conventual orders, relegating the sexually active lay person to a secondary role. Some traditions also propagate the notion that the lay-person should engage in sexual activity only for the purpose of procreation, not as a means of expressing love by giving and receiving pleasure. These ideas have pervaded the thinking of so many genera-tions that they have become part of our social mores, even in a largely secular society, giving rise to unnecessary guilt and an immeasurable amount of unhappiness. That this was not the intention of the great spiritual Masters may be illustrated by Christ's friendship with Mary Magdalene or the many teachings which the Buddha gave to 'house-holders' (i.e. ordinary married people).

The celibate orders hold an honoured place in the tradi-tions of both East and West, but at any point in history only a tiny minority of people will feel called to them. For the rest of humanity sex is, indeed, a fact of life and to those engaged on a quest for personal and spiritual growth this can sometimes feel burdensome because almost all of us have grown up, and still live, in societies where sex has been despiritualised. To reintegrate these two fundamental areas of human experience can be an important step towards wholeness.

The perfume of a flower is closely linked to the sexual life of the plant, and fades as soon as the flower has been pollinated. At the same time it is true that the perfume is the plant's most etherial attribute: it cannot be seen, touched, eaten. It is interesting to note that the German name for essential oil is 'atherische ole' meaning 'etherial oil' and essential oils, sensitively used, can help those who wish to unite the apparent opposites of sex and spirit. We might perhaps start by returning to the first sentence of this chapter and considering the fact that many aphrodisiac oils are also meditation oils. In other words, there is no distinction at a subtle energetic level between meditation and sexual activity.

In practical terms, when using these oils it is perfectly possible to separate the two uses because, as you know, essential oils at a subtle level work according to our intent. If a meditator chooses to work with oil of Sandalwood, and in making that choice focuses on the intent to sit in meditation, it is extremely unlikely that his or her meditation will be disturbed by erotic fantasies provoked by the aphrodisiac action of Sandalwood. Somebody else might choose exactly the same oil for its aphrodisiac effect alone and be delighted with its effectiveness. On the path towards integration, though, we can use such oils in the knowledge that they hold within them both of these possibilities.

Jasmine is perhaps the most important oil for people who wish to spiritualise their sexual relationships. It helps to dispel the fear and guilt that are often associated with sex, so that partners can approach each other truthfully and express through their lovemaking their true nature, which is Divine. At the point of orgasm, self is transcended and with Jasmine we can experience union not only with a sexual partner, but with God.

If your personal belief system precludes the use of the word God, you could substitute 'the Divine', 'the Highest' or whatever expression is meaningful for you. The words we use do not matter; what is important is the integration of sex and spirit.

Although Jasmine is generally acknowledged as a powerful aphrodisiac it is not generally thought of as a meditation oil, however, its more spiritualising properties were known in very ancient times but have been forgotten. At the present time, when so many people are working towards wholeness and spiritual growth, this ancient knowledge is being re-discovered.

Rose and Neroli can be thought of in much the same way since both are aphrodisiacs, albeit less powerful than Jasmine but neither are generally considered as meditation oils. Both of these oils, though, invoke very profound spiritual qualities.

Neroli has the ability to bring us into closer contact with our highest nature and, indeed with the Divine. The orange blossom from which it is distilled has long been regarded as a symbol of purity and the teaching which Neroli embodies is that sexuality is neither pure nor impure. Once we have accepted that sex is not 'dirty' it becomes possible to experience it as an expression of our highest self.

The Rose has always been considered the Flower of Love. To the Greeks of classical antiquity, the Rose was the flower of Aphrodite (Venus), goddess of love, beauty, the arts and creativity in all its forms, although she is most often thought of today as the embodiment of 'profane' love. In early Christian mysticism, though, the Rose was the flower of the Blessed Virgin, symbolising chastity and union with the Holy Spirit. So in the symbolism of the Rose we can see these two apparent opposites brought together: the archetypes of Madonna and Whore are united. The flower and its oil invoke love, whatever form of expression love takes.

The same is true if we look at Rose oil in connection with Chakra energy: Rose has a special affinity with the Heart Chakra, centre of loving energy, which can be expressed as limited, human love or all-embracing Universal Love. Rose also strongly influences the Second Chakra, centre of sexual and creative energy.

Rose helps us to feel more deeply the creative potential of our relationships and brings a gentleness of spirit to sexual expression. The lesson that Rose brings to us is that lovemaking really is about love.

Although these four – Jasmine, Neroli, Rose and Sandalwood – are perhaps the most important in helping to bring human sexuality and spirituality closer together, there are several other oils which do not deserve to be overlooked.

Vetivert, with its ability to balance the energy of the upper and lower chakras is another that unifies the spiritual and physical aspects of human life and so can deepen and enrich sexual relationships.

Rosewood, connecting with the Crown Chakra, can help us become more open to the Divine. Many people find its rich aroma aphrodisiac, and for those who do this oil can make sex a true expression of the higher self.

Patchouli is useful for people who are reluctant to acknowledge their own sexuality, because they feel (maybe unconsciously) that to give physical expression to their emotions is in some way unworthy of their spiritual aspirations. Patchouli grounds us firmly in our physical bodies. It is helpful, too, for people who have difficulty in relationships because they 'live in their heads' and feel somewhat detached from their bodies.

Any of these oils can be used by putting a few drops in a bath before going to bed, and their effect can be prolonged by using the same oil in a burner in the bedroom.

It is important to realise that these oils, and indeed the whole question of sexuality and spirituality, have as much relevance for people who do not have a sexual partner as for those who do. To be ill at ease about one's own sexual feelings can create as much unhappiness outside partnerships as within, and stops many people from forming satisfactory relationships in the long term. Even people who have made a conscious decision that they do not wish to enter a sexual relationship, either for the time being or in the long term, need to acknowledge and accept their own basic sexuality, even though they do not wish to give it outward expression. Using a drop of pure essential oil directly on the skin as a perfume or anointing oil is more suitable than baths and burners for people who are not in a current relationship.

It would be dishonest to pretend that essential oils *alone* are able to bring about such major changes. They must always be used in conjunction with meditation, visualization, affirmations or whatever form of inner work is right for the individual. For some people workshops or individual therapy will be appropriate. What the essential oils do is to facilitate such work.

Of the various oils mentioned in this chapter the three flower absolutes, Jasmine, Neroli and Rose are perhaps the most appropriate for such inner work though the choice of oil must always lie with the person who is going to use it, and if any of the other oils mentioned feel more suitable then they should be used instead.

Here are three meditations, each associated with one of the flower absolutes.

A Neroli Meditation

Place a single drop of Neroli on a handkerchief and inhale it deeply. As you do so, phrase the thought 'Every part of my body is holy'. Place the handkerchief where you can still smell it while you meditate. Spend a few minutes simply focusing on your breath in order to centre the mind and still all 'mental chatter'. Now focus your attention on your physical body, starting with the top of your head.

With your inner eye, examine the colour and texture of your hair, all the features of your face, the softness of your facial skin. Go inside your head and marvel at the miracle which is the human brain and as you move around the body in your meditation, be aware of the network of nerve fibres which connect this wonderful brain to every part of you.

Bring your awareness to the torso, again starting from the outer surface; the skin, the firmness of the ribs lying beneath the skin, the softness of the breasts, if you are a woman. Be aware of your arms, linked to your torso at the shoulder joints, and of your hands, with which we give and receive. Go inside the ribcage and travel around the heart and lungs, working ceaselessly every second of our life on Earth. Look at the great veins and arteries carrying blood to and from your heart, and as you continue to travel around the body, see all the smaller and still smaller vessels that carry that blood to every particle of your body.

Move below the ribcage and be aware of your stomach, liver, gallbladder which make it possible for you to take in and digest your daily food. Move down again to the level of the navel, and feel the difference between the soft belly and strong bones of the hips and lower back. Go inside your belly and make friends with your intestines, for it is here that all the nutrients from digested food are absorbed in a form that can nourish your whole body.

Now focus on your genitals, becoming aware of their wonderful design. Consider their outer surfaces, the shapes, forms, colour and texture. Go gently within the testes, or to the ovaries and the heart of the womb and consider their intricate mechanisms and their potential for creating new life.

Finally, focus on your legs and your feet. Look inside at the long, straight bones that support you and the strong muscles that carry you forward. Consider how your feet connect you to the supporting Earth.

Now ask yourself 'Is any part of my body separate from the rest? Is there any part of my body that is not nourished by my blood and linked to my brain? Can any part of my body exist independently from the whole? Whereabouts in this miraculous human body does my soul reside?'

Compare your body now with the orange tree. Think of

the roots, the trunk, sap and bark, the leaves and twigs, the buds and flowers and the round, juicy fruit. Consider especially the white flowers, and their perfume – the spiritual emanation of the tree, and ask yourself 'Can the flower grow without the root? Can the fruit form unless the flower is fertilised?'

Bring your awareness gradually back to the place where you are sitting. Take up your handkerchief so that you can inhale another deep breath of Neroli and say to yourself once again 'Every part of my body is holy. I am whole'.

A Jasmine Meditation

Begin in the same way as for the Neroli meditation, except that you will place on your handkerchief a single drop of Jasmine.

When you have centred yourself, allow a picture of the person you love to form in your mind's eye. See your beloved first clothed, and then unclothed, and contemplate this body that is so dear to you.

As you do so, imagine a beam of silver light illuminating your beloved. As you watch, the light is absorbed into your lover's body until it has become a body of silver light. Experience the love that you feel for this radiant being.

Now the same beam of silver light shines on yourself, and you feel it pervading every pore, every cell of your body. You and your beloved become alike in your radiance. Now your two bodies of light merge totally with one another. You have become one being, of a brightness that is almost beyond human imagining.

Stay with your awareness of that union and that brightness for a while. When you feel ready, bring your awareness very gently back to the place where you are sitting, but be aware that you can carry the silver body within you, that you and your beloved are radiant beings of light at all times.

Inhale deeply from the Jasmine oil to anchor this knowledge in your heart.

A Rose Meditation

Once again, you begin the meditation by breathing deeply the aroma of the Rose.

When you feel still and centred, allow a picture of the person you love to appear sitting in front of you. From your Heart Centre a beam of rose-coloured light connects to the Heart Centre of your beloved making the base of a triangle, and from each of your hearts another beam connects to a point above your heads.

Feel now that you are being drawn up the beam of light towards the point at the top of the triangle. At the same time your beloved is being drawn up to the same place. Here, your higher selves meet and are united.

In the centre of the space formed by your triangle of light, allow a symbol to appear which represents the union of your higher selves. Draw this symbol towards yourself and into your Heart Centre. Feel it expanding so that it completely fills your heart and then your entire body. Now allow the symbol to be drawn into the Heart centre of your beloved. Such is the abundance of love contained within the symbol that you remain entirely filled by it even as it expands to fill the heart and body of your beloved. Love fills the whole of the space formed by your triangle of light, and continues to expand until you feel it could fill the entire Universe, for what you are experiencing is Universal Love.

Stay with that knowledge for a little time, until you feel ready to gently return your awareness to the place where you are sitting. Take a few deep breaths of your Rose absolute to help anchor the beauty of this meditation in your heart.

The Neroli meditation is for anyone, whether in a relationship or not. The Jasmine and Rose meditations are, clearly, for people who are in a current relationship, although it is not necessary for both to be physically present: you can do these meditations even if you are separated from the person you love by thousands of miles. In fact, such meditations become very valuable during times of separation, especially if both partners know that the other is doing a similar meditation.

If you are not separated by distance, it is very beautiful to sit together for these meditations. Sit facing each other a little distance apart. It can reinforce the feeling of connectedness if you share your flower absolute by inhaling deeply from it and then silently handing the handkerchief to your partner at the beginning and at the end of the meditation.

If you genuinely desire to spiritualize your sexual relationship sitting together in meditation (whether the ones I have outlined or any other form) is a powerful way to do so. If your partner is unwilling to sit and meditate with you, it may be that you need to ask yourself whether you are with the right partner.

Finally, to return to the subject of celibacy mentioned at the beginning of this chapter: in the present century so much emphasis has been placed on the importance of a fulfilling love-life that there is a temptation to regard celibacy as an impoverished state of being, or even an unhealthy one. There is an irony in this reversal of the outlook of earlier centuries. A person who leads a celibate life unwillingly may well feel impoverished but for those who have consciously chosen celibacy this is not necessarily true. A celibate life is neither better nor worse than a life that includes sexual activity.

There are essential oils that will support those who have made this choice as well as those who feel they have been pushed into it unwillingly. Marjoram is comforting and anti-aphrodisiac for those who would like to be in a relationship but are not for whatever reason and for people who have been bereaved or otherwise separated from a loved partner.

It eases loneliness and offers emotional warmth. It is probably most effective when used in evening baths. Lavender, with its aura of cleanliness and simplicity lends itself to those who have chosen to be celibate. Simply inhaling it enhances and reinforces that decision.

So let us be thankful to the bountiful Universe for providing such a wealth of plants and essential oils on our planet that every individual can find among them the right ones for such diverse needs.

CHAPTER 13

Entering Earthly Life

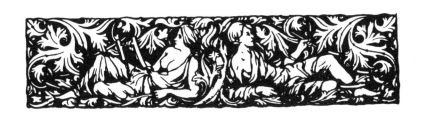

Much has been written about the physical benefits to the mother of using essential oils in pregnancy and childbirth, but little about the use of Subtle Aromatherapy during this very special time. Bringing a new person into being is both an awesome responsibility and a source of great joy. Sometimes, though, the responsibility, fear and other emotions make it difficult to experience the joy, and here sensitive use of essential oils can support the future parents and help to restore a sense of joyful anticipation.

Subtle Aromatherapy is particularly well fitted to the needs of a pregnant woman. The very tiny quantities of oil used and the gentle methods of applying them make it a safe form of therapy from the physical point of view, while the emotional/spiritual properties of the oils resonate with the heightened awareness that characterises pregnancy.

The range of oils that can be used is fairly restricted, as it must exclude all those that could pose any danger to the mother or her unborn child. You will find warnings about potentially harmful oils among the entries towards the end of this book. If you want to use any oil not included here, do check its safety in a good book on traditional aromatherapy. In particular, avoid oils described as emmenagogue during the first 4/5 months, as they can induce bleeding.

Fortunately, the oils that can be regarded as safe are the ones which embody the subtle vibrations most appropriate to pregnancy. As you might expect, they include the delicate floral absolutes of Neroli and Rose (but not Jasmine), Lavender, Mandarin and English or Roman Camomiles (Anthemis nobilis), NOT 'Blue Camomile', a name often used to describe Artemisia arborescens, which is a powerful emmenagogue. Camomile, Lavender and Rose are all traditionally listed as emmenagogues, but the risk with them is minuscule when used in Subtle Aromatherapy applications. I would suggest avoiding them only if there is a previous history of miscarriage. The vibrational quality of

Rose, in particular, is so fitted to the condition of mother-hood that it would be a great pity to forgo it.

Rose speaks, above all, of love: the love of the couple who have come together to make this child, their love for the baby, and the love the baby will eventually share with them. Mandarin is a particularly lovely oil to use during pregnancy because it has an open, childlike quality and invokes happiness, and Neroli reflects the purity of a new-born child. These two oils can be used from the earliest moments to the end of pregnancy. The baby, too, will benefit from being surrounded by fragrance during its time of waiting in the womb. It is known that babies perceive aromas long before birth and, when born, can recognize perfumes used by their mothers while carrying them.

The father of the unborn child may often be overlooked to some extent as his partner becomes the focus of attention, but he, too, deserves the pleasure of using fragrant oils. Burners around the home mean that both parents can share the enjoyment, and the vibrational influence, of the same oil.

As the time of birth approaches, it is good to include some oils in the preparations for the baby's arrival. I am not speaking here of oils to facilitate labour, which belong more properly to traditional aromatherapy, but oils to welcome the child with fragrance. Choose one of the oils that the mother has been using during her pregnancy and place one single drop on the cloth that is to be wrapped round the baby as soon as it is delivered, and another drop on the sheet lining the cradle. Have the same oil to hand for the baby's first bath, and add to it one drop of essential oil mixed in a teaspoon of almond or grapeseed oil. (Never use essential oils undiluted for babies.)

Surrounding the newborn infant with fragrance in this way eases the shock of entering this physical world. The best oil for this purpose is Neroli, especially if the mother has been using it beforehand, though Rose or Mandarin are almost as lovely.

Some parents wish to welcome the incoming soul before it enters the outer world or even to invite a soul into their lives, so here is a meditation that can be used at three special times: as soon as the mother knows that she has conceived, at the time of the baby's first movements or when a couple wish to conceive, to draw a soul towards them.

A MEDITATION TO WELCOME THE INCOMING SOUL

The couple should sit down facing each other in a space that they have made as beautiful as they can, with some fresh flowers – Roses if possible – and candlelight. Before sitting to meditate, they should prepare some oil in a small dish by mixing two drops of Rose absolute into two teaspoons of almond or grapeseed oil and placing the dish between them when they sit. The dish should preferably be beautiful to look at, of delicate china, glass or crystal.

Dipping their fingers into the oil, each in turn anoints the other first on the forehead, then at the Heart Chakra, next on the belly a little below the navel, and finally on the palm of each hand. At the Brow Chakra this is done with the intent of focusing thought upon the child-to-be, at the Heart with the intent of offering that child love, on the belly with the intent of nurturing the child and on the hands with the intent of welcoming the child into this world. The intentions can be voiced aloud, or held in the mind. During the rest of the meditation the couple may either sit holding both hands, or the man may place one hand on the woman's belly. This is particularly appropriate if the meditation is to mark their baby's first movements within the womb.

Now each sees a beam of rose-coloured light joining their

Heart Chakras to form the base of a triangle and another from each of their Heart Chakras joining to form the apex of the triangle above their heads. Slowly, they feel themselves drawn up to the top of the triangle, and into this space they invite the incoming soul. From the depth of their hearts they speak to this being of the love they feel for it already, their desire to welcome this soul into their lives and their intent to nurture and care for it. They remain for some time with these feelings of great love and happiness before slowly and gently returning their awareness to the present time and the place where they are sitting.

CHAPTER 14

The Great Transition

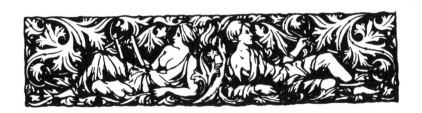

At the major time of transition which we call death, Subtle Aromatherapy can be a comfort and support to both the dying person and to family, friends and carers. The subtle, indeed spiritual, aspects of aromatherapy become even more important when physical treatment is no longer appropriate. Aromatherapists engaged in hospice work repeatedly tell of the tranquillity, acceptance, even joy which sensitively-chosen essential oils have been able to bring to the people in their care.

A considerable number of aromatherapists now work as volunteers in hospices and it is clear from discussing this work with some of them that they are practising Subtle Aromatherapy, even if they have never come across that concept before. The nature of their patients' illness usually obliges them to use extremely low dilutions of essential oil, and to massage with only the lightest of touch, if at all. Many of them speak of the great pleasure a drop of oil on a handkerchief has given to people too frail to want even a gentle hand massage. Above all, it is the therapists' attitudes and expectations that have lifted their work onto an altogether higher plane: having no prospect of physical 'cure' in mind, they devote themselves to the relief of pain and, beyond that, to the mental, emotional and spiritual wellbeing of the people they care for. As I have emphasised throughout this book, the intent and thought of the therapist are central factors in all subtle or vibrational healing.

I have myself been privileged to work with only two people who were terminally ill, but both of these encounters were times of deep learning for me, as well as confirming all that I had been told by my colleagues who do such work all the time.

At this point, it may be fruitful to examine the concept of healing. There is a widespread misconception that to 'heal' means to 'cure' in the sense of making the physical body well. This view of healing leads to the idea that the healer has failed if the person they have been working with dies, whereas to help a person to approach death consciously, calmly and without fear is perhaps the greatest gift that a healer can offer.

The word 'heal' is of ancient origin, and it shares it roots with the words 'holy' and 'whole' as well as 'hale' and 'healthy'. When both the healer and the person in need of healing let go of the desire to make healthy, the deeper healing, the making holy, can begin.

Part of the value of Subtle Aromatherapy in such healing is the power of essential oils to touch the mind and spirit in ways that can seldom be expressed in words. Oils which bring the user into closer contact with the higher self and with the Divine are the first that come to mind, together with those that ease times of change and loss.

Frankincense connects us with our Higher Self which is eternal and holy and makes it easier to let go of earthly attachments. Cedarwood strengthens our connection with the Divine and Angelica opens our awareness of the angelic realm. All three of these oils speak to the soul, helping it to loose its ties with the earthly body it has inhabited for a span.

Cypress eases all times of transition – puberty, career changes, marriage, divorce or religious conversion as well as dying. From that aspect it might be compared to the Dr. Bach Flower Remedy Walnut and some people benefit from using both together. It has also been associated with the time of death for many thousands of years and the tree is often planted in cemeteries. The flame-like shape of the tree leads our thoughts and aspirations ever higher and its evergreen or ever-living foliage carries a message of life eternal. Rosewood and Neroli both relate to the crown Chakra and strengthen spirituality. Rosewood in particular can bring about an opening of this chakra. In fact, with many people there is a spontaneous opening of this chakra as death approaches, but Rosewood may facilitate this.

Two oils which are frequently mentioned by hospice workers as giving great pleasure to their patients are Bergamot and Rose. Both of these oils have an affinity with the Heart Chakra, and the fact that they are among the most beautiful aromas in the whole repertoire is not insignificant. Perfume is the most etherial, the least tangible of sensory pleasures, which can still give pleasure to a person so ill that most earthly delights are denied them. Bergamot, in particular, helps if the chakra is closed because of grief. This is a sunny oil: it assuages grief and brings light into the darkest situation. It is often described as uplifting, and in the context of dying, this quality of the oil is enhanced and refined, so it truly lifts the soul upwards towards the Light.

Rose also allays grief, bringing comfort and consolation. Rose is associated not only with human love, but with Universal Love. It offers solace to relatives and friends as well as the dying person. The Heart Chakra is the centre of devotion to the Deity, which is often very strong in the days preceding death. The element of aesthetic pleasure is very great with this oil too. Heat alters the delicate aroma, so it is not wise to use Rose in burners. Put a drop on a handkerchief to be smelt from time to time.

However, the one oil above all others which seems to be of supreme help to both the dying and those around them is Melissa. This oil, too, is an aid in all times of transition but it has particular significance at the end of earthly life. It seems to dispel fear and bring about acceptance at the approach of death. It eases shock, particularly if somebody has died suddenly or violently, such as in a road accident. Melissa has affinities not only with the Heart Chakra but the Solar Plexus, the centre of expression of the will. It helps to align the human will with the Divine will, and this can make approaching death easier to accept, both for the dying person and for those who know they will soon be left behind.

Several experiences suggest that Melissa helps us to remember past lives, and I often think that is one reason why it is so comforting to the dying: by reminding us that we have lived before, it helps us to understand that we will live again.

In connection with this, it is of the utmost importance that therapists who work with the terminally ill respect their views and beliefs. If the therapist believes, for example, in the possibility of rebirth in a new body, while the dying person believes in an eternal life in heaven, or thinks that physical death is the end of all existence, it is paramount that the therapist should say nothing that contradicts that belief. Let the essential oils speak for themselves. They connect with the highest level of mind where words become meaningless. If Cypress or Melissa evoke a consciousness of eternal life, each person smelling them will bring to that consciousness their own understanding of what is meant by eternal life.

In working with people who are dying, the methods for using essential oils are fairly limited: massage will probably have to be restricted to hands, feet or face, baths may not be possible so the use of burners, simple inhaling and anointing become very important. In fact these methods are also those which are the most subtle in their effect, which makes them all the more suitable for use at this time. Having said that, I would also say that as long as any form of massage is possible, it should be offered. A great deal of work in hospitals and hospices has shown how much comfort and benefit gentle touch can give and it would be a shame to deny it as long as it is enjoyed.

Burners in the room are a simple method, and can easily be used by nursing staff or relatives if the aromatherapist provides some suitable oils and instructions. The final choice of oil must, of course, be the one that is most enjoyed, or asked for at any specific time, by the ill person, and if it is not one that figures in the preceding notes, that does not matter at all – they are merely a summary of those I believe most likely to help.

Anointing, by simply putting a little oil directly on the skin, is a beautiful way to use essential oils, carrying with it certain sacramental connotations (though the aromatherapist must never usurp the role of the priest or other spiritual leader). Oils can be gently placed on hands or forehead, but it is important to remember that they should be well diluted, as illness and drug side-effects often leave the skin extremely fragile.

The simplest method of all is just to put a drop of oil on a handkerchief or tissue, and this is often enjoyed very much by a sick person because they are in control of when they choose to smell it.

The family and friends of a dying person need loving and healing, too, though very often they are reticent about asking for any help. They feel that their needs are secondary to those of their dying friend, that they must not appear to grieve, or do anything that could be interpreted as weakness. A friend who nursed her dying husband at home until very near the end of his life, would only ask me for an aromatherapy session if she had strained her back lifting him, or had some other physical injury. Only then could she 'allow' her self to seek help.

Sometimes a person who is ready to die, is held back by the reluctance of family and friends to let go of them. They may try to maintain an atmosphere of cheerfulness at all times which can, in fact, be very stressful for themselves and their loved one. It can prevent the sharing of deep emotions, and even the settling of practical matters. Relatives often find it very difficult to talk about what will happen after somebody has died, whereas the dying person might really want to discuss subjects as variable as the funeral arrangements, their children's education or their feelings about the possibility of a spouse re-marrying at some time in the future. It is often easier to make a peaceful transition from this life when such thoughts and feelings have been honestly and openly shared.

Communication can sometimes be eased when an oil burner is used in the patient's room. An oil which is softening and opening (Bergamot or Rosewood, perhaps) can exert its gentle influence on everybody who spends any time in the room. It is good to ask a close relative to be responsible for lighting a burner regularly, or putting some oil on a hankie between the aromatherapist's visits to ensure that the oils are in fairly continuous use.

If you have been in close contact with a dying person's family and friends in the time leading up to their death, they may well turn to you for support and comfort when death eventually takes place. Their need might be for a hug or somebody to talk to but if you do have an opportunity to offer an aromatherapy treatment it could be of enormous help.

In the immediate aftermath of bereavement, I think that simple, physical massage is usually the most appropriate form of treatment. If somebody had died at home, or has entered a hospital or hospice only a short time before dying, the close relatives will also probably have been the chief carers and may have had weeks or months of broken nights, lifting, washing, feeding and caring for an otherwise helpless person. They are likely to have ignored or denied their own fatigue throughout this time, and struggled to maintain an appearance of strength. Once the need for this has disappeared, exhaustion engulfs them. When somebody dies after being in hospital or a hospice for a long time, those closest to them will probably have been travelling daily to visit, maybe sitting up all night at the bedside towards the end, and are also likely to be in a state of total fatigue, as well as the inevitable grief and distress.

Relief from physical aches and the comfort of a human touch become very important then. At the same time, the therapist should bear in mind the subtle attributes of the essential oils and choose perhaps Melissa, Rose or Bergamot for the great comfort they can give at a less tangible level. Rose is particularly indicated for those who find themselves unable to express their grief openly. Grief closes the Heart Chakra, Rose tends to open it and often, a very gentle massage with Rose oil releases unshed tears. These tears are healing. If you encounter this reaction, allow the person to cry for as long as they need to, offering tissues, a warm drink or a hug only when you will not intrude on their grief. Some may want to continue the massage, others will not.

A bereaved person often needs to talk, and it helps to talk to somebody outside their family and immediate circle. The same kind of release that allows tears to flow during or after a massage will often unleash a torrent of words. Some aromatherapists feel well able to deal with such a situation, feeling indeed that listening is part of their relationship with their clients. Even so, I would suggest contacting a trained bereavement counsellor who will have a special understanding of the confused feelings that many people experience when somebody very close to them has died. They may feel relief, guilt and anger as well as grief. If somebody has been ill for a long time, in great pain, needing constant attention, it is often a relief when that person dies, but those closest to them feel extremely guilty about experiencing relief. A bereaved person may feel angry at their partner for leaving them, guilty about not preventing the death (even though it was entirely beyond their ability to do so) and totally at a loss to understand their own reaction. A counsellor who works frequently with bereaved people will be able to reassure them that all these emotions are normal, permissible and need to be expressed.

An aromatherapist in an ordinary practice will not often

work with people who are terminally ill, but is more likely to see people who need support and comfort after a relative or close friend has died, so these aspects are particularly relevant if you work in a clinic, salon or health centre as opposed to (or, indeed, as well as) doing voluntary work in a hospice.

Finally, we must not forget the emotional and spiritual needs of therapists who work with the dying. They may find themselves having to confront emotions such as their feelings about their own death, memories of somebody they have lost, fears about the death of people close to them. Terminally ill people may be emaciated or bloated by drug side-effects, or badly disfigured by surgery, and therapists who work with them might find that this raises issues about their own bodies. Then, of course, there will inevitably be some distress when a patient dies, even though it has been anticipated.

The question of 'Who cares for the carers?' arises and such care is not always available. Peer support is often the only possibility. Fortunately, therapists can always benefit from the oils that they use to help others. Much of the time, they will be inhaling uplifting, spiritualizing oils while they are working but it is important to remember such things as closing the chakras before working, and using cleansing and purifying oils in baths. Otherwise there is the danger of becoming drained and exhausted at the subtle energetic level.

Not everybody feels able to engage in such work, but those who do almost always find that it becomes an important part of their own spiritual growth. And what greater service can any of us give to our fellow humans than enriching the final days of earthly life.

Whether or not we choose to work among terminally ill people, each one of us must come face to face with death, if only at the end of our own lives. Almost everybody will at some point in their lives be left to grieve the death of somebody close, so I would like to close this chapter by offering for your consideration a meditation for such times.

MEDITATION FOR A DEAD FRIEND

Let those who have been closest to a person during life come together as soon as possible after their friend has died. Prepare the room by putting two or three drops of true Melissa oil in a burner, and if any of the participants have Lemon Balm growing in a garden, it is good to pick some and place bunches of the fresh herb in the room.

Sitting in a circle, place a crystal in the centre. A clear quartz crystal would be best. Spend a few moments breathing quietly to calm and centre the energy of the group. Let each person hold a mental picture of the friend who has left this earthly life.

Now, everyone in the circle imagines a shaft of white light joining his or her Heart Chakra to that of the person on the left, and another joining it to the crystal.

Allow love to pour forth from each Heart Chakra, filling the circle with pure, loving energy. Feel the love increasing until the circle can no longer contain it. At this point, envisage all your love focused by the crystal into an immense beam of white light shining upwards.

See the friend that you all loved standing in the centre of this light. Watch the light increasing in intensity and pervading the body of your friend until it is totally transmuted into light. Slowly, you see this radiant Being, who was once your earthly friend, ascending the great shaft of light until it is lost to your view.

As your friend is lost to your sight, hold in your heart the knowledge that every one of us is just such a radiant Being, even when the radiance is clouded by a body of flesh, and that nothing divides us from those who are no longer burdened by such a body.

CHAPTER 15

Healing our Planet

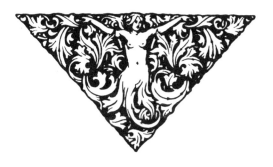

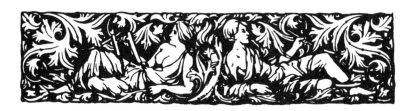

Y ou may feel, as I do, that it is of limited use to heal
ourselves or others without caring for the planet on
which we live.

Our good Planet Earth, who we may also call Gaia, or the
Earth Mother, is deeply wounded. We have plundered her
treasures, poisoned her seas and rivers, polluted her air, and
damaged the protective mantle that enables us to live safely
on her surface. For too long men have thought of her as an
inert collection of rocks and minerals from which they could
draw indefinitely and into which they could dump all manner
of waste.

The scientist James Lovelock touched a chord in many
hearts when he proposed the idea that the Earth is a living
organism, and took the name of Gaia, the primordial Earth
Mother, from ancient myth to describe her.

Our Mother is wounded, but we depend on her totally to
sustain us. Unless we heal our Mother we will not survive.

I think that few people reading this are unaware of these
facts, but I would like to share with you some of the
environmental and planetary healing possibilities inherent in
the use of essential oils. Plants connect us in a real and
tangible way with the Earth, and we should never lose sight of
the fact that our essential oils are made in the cells of plants.

Planetary healing, like all other forms of healing, can be
accomplished on many different levels, and the need is so
great, the time so short, that to be sure of success we need to
work in every way available to us as individuals to bring this
about. No single individual can heal the whole Earth alone
but every single individual is needed to accomplish this.

We can work towards planetary healing physically,
mentally and in subtle ways.

At the physical level, we can 'walk gently on the Earth', in
other words, live our lives in such a way that we take as little
as possible from the Earth's resources and add as little as
possible to the total load of pollution. To do this may entail

changing the way we heat our homes, the cleaning and other products we use in them, the materials used to make our furniture and household equipment, the clothes we wear, cosmetics, toiletries and other personal products, our method of transport, the ways we dispose of waste and even the food we eat. Do not be tempted to think that the little you can do is too small to have any effect: remember 'If you are not part of the solution, you are part of the problem'.

Essential oils can contribute to our efforts at the physical level by replacing many synthetically produced items: perfumes, skincare products, bath additives, personal hygiene products, domestic disinfectants, air fresheners, insect repellents and even synthetic drugs. In addition, many of the environment-friendly household and personal products on sale are perfumed with essential oils and other plant extracts, rather than the synthetic perfumes commonly found in such items. Others are perfume-free and you can, if you wish, add essentials oils to them to enhance your personal environment.

Another important factor is to use only essential oils produced without the use of chemicals, i.e. organically grown or collected from wild plants. The growing of aromatics for essential oil production may amount to only a minute part of world agriculture but here, as with our personal and household consumption, each small contribution to the health of the planet is significant.

Organic growers care for the soil as well as for their plants – not using chemicals is only one part of the story – and they put rotted vegetable matter (compost) back into the soil to replace the nutrients which each harvest of plants has taken out. This maintains the structure of the soil, as well as its stock of nutrients and in this way they help to constantly renew Earth's precious mantle. This is in sharp contrast to chemical agriculture which uses chemical fertilisers to increase crop yields, but does not put any organic matter back into the soil to maintain its texture. Eventually this leads to a breaking down of the soil, erosion and the dust-bowl phenomenon.

At the mental level, we can work by talking to friends, writing to newspapers, joining local, national and international pressure groups and charities, for the poisoned river thousands of miles away matters every bit as much as the toxic waste dump near your home.

At the subtle level there is much that we can do to bring about environmental and planetary healing, using essential oils, crystals, meditation and visualization.

Working in this way, we need to start with our homes and immediate surroundings just as with work on the physical plane. Patterns of negative energy can build up in a house as the result of past events or previous occupants whose dark thought-forms may linger long after they have gone, even such things as old battles fought on the place where your home now stands. Then there are the various factors that contribute to geopathic stress such as negative ley-lines, underground water, mineral deposits and negative earth rays. (These are rays that have become distorted before reaching the Earth's surface.) Because planetary energies have been changing, such negative influences may also shift, and a house which 'felt good' when you first moved into it may acquire quite a dark energy.

Such factors can lead to spiritual or psychic unease, depression, chronic fatigue and ill-health. If you think that your home may be affected in this way, you might try dowsing to locate areas of negativity, as suggested in an earlier chapter, or asking an experienced dowser to do so for you. It is especially important to clear any negative energy that may be found in areas where people spend a lot of time, such as a bedroom, favourite chair or a desk used daily for work, etc.

If you do find that there is some unhelpful energy in the house, especially if it is a negative thought-form, or an emanation from past events, you may well be able to clear it by vapourising appropriate essential oils regularly and performing appropriate visualizations and meditation. Juniper is a particularly helpful oil to use in this context, for its psychic cleansing properties, or you might find Cedar, Lavender, Pine, Rosemary or Eucalyptus appropriate. Stand a burner with a few drops of your chosen oil in the room or area where the negativity is most strongly felt each day for seven days, or more if you feel that it is still needed.

During this time you may wish to dedicate some periods of meditation to the cleansing of the house. Indeed, regular meditation is one of the best ways of clearing negative energies from a building, especially group meditation. If you have fellow-meditators among your friends, you might ask them to join in. In particular, chanting the cosmic sound OM helps to dispel negative thought-forms from an area. The chanting should be kept up for some time – at least 40 minutes if you can manage it – and repeated as often as possible. The support of a group is particularly valuable here, as it become far easier to sustain a long period of chanting when a number of people are taking part. Be sure to burn an appropriate essential oil during the periods of meditation or chanting.

If you like working with crystals, you might prefer to place a single drop of your chosen essential oil or blend on a large crystal and place this in the area that needs to be cleansed, or on several crystals placed at strategic points. If you are uncertain about working with crystals yourself, you might want to ask somebody who is experienced in that field to choose a suitable crystal or crystals and conduct a simple ceremony for you, or you could collaborate in selecting oils and crystals to complement each other.

Crystals are an effective way of neutralising negative energy that is caused by physical factors – geopathic stress – and this is an area in which essential oils alone are not much help. If you think that you (or your clients or friends) are affected by geopathic stress I would strongly advise asking an experienced crystal healer to help. Alternatively, you can buy a small device called a RadiTech that plugs into an electrical circuit to neutralise such energies. Whichever method you decide upon, it would be good to also burn some essential oils in the area.

After any such cleansing, it is good to vapourise in the area some essential oils that generate good, positive energy. Depending on the place that has been cleansed, whether it is a bedroom, study, meditation room or general living area, you might choose from among Bergamot, Cedarwood, Lavender, Orange, Neroli, Petitgrain, Rose, Rosewood, Sandalwood or Vetivert in burners or on a crystal and it would be good to do this for seven days, too, though there is no harm at all in using these oils for longer periods. You can also ring the changes among these oils, selecting whichever one appeals to you most at a particular moment. If a whole house has been cleansed, you might choose different oils for various parts of the house.

Moving outwards from the home, at least one spiritual teacher places emphasis on the importance of all healers, meditators and people who are engaged on a spiritual quest, taking responsibility for their immediate environment. Just as environmental activists will tackle issues such as waste dumping, industrial effluent and so on at a local level, the 'spiritual activist' meditates on the local area, perhaps for three to five miles around, and sends healing energy out into the town, village or countryside around. In particular, when doing such meditations, it is good to focus on places where a lot of people congregate together, such as hospitals or the local supermarket. If there is a local trouble-spot, such as a pub, football ground or other place where fighting often occur, or an accident black-spot, it helps to put some pacifying thoughts into that place.

There may be one or more places in your town or village that simply don't 'feel right' and these will benefit from healing meditation, too. It may be that such places coincide with the observable trouble spots, or a study of local history, legends or even gossip may show that the place is associated with dark events in the past, such as the site of a gallows, or a long-forgotten battle but there may not be any identifiable reason why a psychic black-spot exists. Places, like people, can be 'dis-eased' and can be healed in similar ways.

Dowsing a local map can help to locate places in need of healing that you may not be aware of personally. The points where ley-lines cross are always areas of strong energy and this energy is not always beneficial. It can be negative as often as not. Don't rely on the known positions of local ley-lines, unless they have been established very recently, as there have been many changes in the ley-line grid in recent years. Get an experienced dowser to work with a local map, and send healing to the crossover points. Doing this with a map of the town where I live revealed no less than five ley-lines crossing at the point where there had been a disastrous fire, and a crossover of three lines at one of our most dangerous road junctions.

Here is a simple meditation that you can do alone or in a group to heal your local environment:

Choose a healing, cleansing or calming essential oil, depending on what you perceive to be the greatest need of the places you want to heal and put a few drops in a burner. Sit quietly and focus on your breathing, and as you do so, form a mental picture of the place to which you want to send good, healing energy. As you breathe in allow yourself to be very aware of the aroma of the oil being vapourised and feel the healing energy of that oil pervading your body, mind and spirit. As you breathe out, consciously direct healing to the place you have chosen, imagining the healing energy of the essential oil strengthening your intent. As you repeat this with each breath, a real connection with the place that needs healing will be built up.

You can even direct such a meditation towards individuals who seem to present problems in your locality! It may be a local politician, a property developer or the leader of a gang of hooligans. Send healing to such people instead of animosity. Do it regularly, and in a group if possible. You might be surprised at the outcome.

Another way to heal your environment is to focus on some special place that seems to generate good, positive energy and meditate with the intent of spreading this positive energy throughout the area. In many places, there are already groups of people linked to Fountain International who use this form of meditation. They choose a focal point in their area, which they describe as the 'hara' of the district (hara being another term for the Second Chakra) on which all members meditate individually, as well as meeting for talks and meditations.

The meditation that I have described for healing your immediate locality can equally well be used to heal needy places throughout the world. Breathing and using the energy of the essential oil in just the same way, focus upon and send your healing thoughts out to areas of conflict or unrest, famine, drought, earthquake or other natural or man-made disasters.

Above all, though, we need to express our love and our intent to heal the harm that has already been done to the whole planet, as well as doing everything in our power to prevent further harm.

Here are two meditations for planetary healing that I would like to share with you. As always, before you begin chose an essential oil that will enhance and strengthen your meditation. The oil that I use most often for these meditations is Rosewood. As well as its properties as a meditation aid, this oil holds special significance in relation to planetary healing because the tree from which it is distilled grows only in the

Amazon rain forests. Destruction of the rain forests threatens the trees, and without them there would be no more oil of Rosewood, so it seems fitting to take this oil as a symbol of the many threatened ecosystems, and of the Earth Mother herself. Of course, if any other oil holds special significance for you in relation to the healing of the planet, you should use that oil, for it will strengthen your meditation more than merely following my suggestions.

The first meditation is similar to that for healing your home environment, for indeed the planet is your home.

Place your burner with the essential oil, or a crystal on which you have put one drop of the oil, or simply a handkerchief with a drop of oil, where you can smell it when you sit to meditate. As with all meditations, sit quietly for a few moments and focus on your breath. Now allow a picture of the planet to form in your mind's eye, and imagine that you are able to hold the Earth in your hands. Depending on your imagination and your temperament, you may wish to do this by seeing the planet as very small, or by feeling or seeing yourself expand to a tremendous size, so that you are able to hold the whole of the actual planet.

With great love, and with reverence for the miracle that is the Planet Earth, turn the globe carefully around and around in your hands. Feel the many different textures of its surface, the rough, hard mountains, the soft sands, gentle forests and prairies. Feel the heat around the equator and the cold around the Poles. Look at the many different colours that make up this wonderful ball. Look at the sparkling waters that cover so much of it. Marvel at all the different kinds of creatures that live upon it.

As you continue to turn the globe around, become aware of the many wounds that show on its surface: see the areas of drought, the trees poisoned by acid rain, the shrinking forests, the thick haze of pollution, the contaminated oceans and the shores covered in oil. See the suffering of animals that have lost their habitat, the people who are starving. Throughout this meditation, draw in healing energy from the essential oil with every in-breath, and on every out-breath send healing to each part of the planet that is in need of it.

At the completion of the meditation, see yourself and the Earth returned to their true size, and give thanks for the existence of this planet.

The second meditation is one of optimism and assurance, which we sometimes need to counteract the messages of doom and gloom and the people who tell us it is already too late. It is very easy to become discouraged and feel that nothing we can do personally will make any difference to the eventual fate of the planet, but remember that 'thought precedes form' and the more negative thoughts we hold concerning the possible destruction of the planet as we know it, the more chance there is of that coming to pass. Conversely, the conviction that our efforts DO count can encourage us to try even harder. So, here is a joyful meditation! For this meditation, use an uplifting essential oil such as Bergamot or Orange. If you have Grapefruit oil, that would be even better, for as well as having the cheerful, uplifting qualities of all the citrus oils, Grapefruit connects us strongly with Gaia.

Seated comfortably, focus quietly on your breath for a few minutes, savouring the aroma of your chosen oil. Now imagine that your chair or cushion is fading away and that you are supported on a feathery cloud. On your cloud, you float higher and higher above the world, until you can see the whole of Earth turning in space. But this is a very special cloud that can carry you through time as well as space, and soon you are looking down on the Earth 50 years from now, 100 years from now, 300 years from now. At this point in time, your cloud carries you down closer to the Earth's surface, and you can see in detail the forests and plains, the rivers and oceans, and you see that the forests are thriving, the plains are green and the seas and rivers sparkling and teeming with life. The cloud carries you up and onwards in time again, 1,000 years into the future and again you move closer to the surface so that you can see all that is taking place on the planet. You see a green and fertile Earth, the thick smogs of polluted air are nowhere to be seen, the deep scars that industry and warfare had inflicted on her have healed and new life grown over them. You see no signs of conflict or suffering, mankind is living at peace with his fellow-beings, and with the Earth that supports all life.

Gradually your cloud transports you back through time and space. You become conscious once more of being supported by your chair or cushion. Focus on the aroma of the essential oil and allow it to remind you where you are as you bring your awareness back to the present time and place. Before you open your eyes, place in your heart the image of a beautiful, peaceful Earth, an Earth that has one again been made whole, serenely turning through space far, far into the future. Hold this image always as a focus for all your planetary healing work.

CHAPTER 16

The Subtle
Properties of
Individual Oils

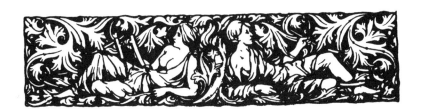

Angelica
Angelica archangelica

This oil, as its name suggests, helps to make the user more open to angelic energies. For some, this may mean actual encounters with angels, angelic visions or messages from angels, or, without seeing or hearing anything, one may have a strong impression of a benevolent presence. For others, it may mean being more in tune with their higher selves. The plant is often referred to in mediaeval and Renaissance herbals as Archangels, Angels' Herb or the Herb of the Holy Spirit. You may find it stated in textbooks that these names were given to the plant because of its almost miraculous powers of healing at a physical level, particularly during the epidemics of plague that repeatedly swept across Europe. These healing properties are very real and we can draw on them in both subtle and traditional aromatherapy. All the same, I think it unlikely that those mediaeval writers did not know the spiritual attributes of this plant.

The oil most usually used is extracted from the root (though there is also an oil obtained from the seeds) and like many root oils is very grounding in nature. If this seems contradictory, consider how necessary it is for visionaries, channels and spiritual seekers to remain well grounded in their human bodies if they are to function in the everyday world.

The living Angelica plant speaks to us eloquently of this necessity. Underground it forms strong and solid roots, above-ground the whole plant seems to aspire heavenwards: the powerful stems soar to two metres in height, topped by a mass of delicate greenish-white flowers so etherial in appearance as to seem almost insubstantial.

The aroma, somewhat overpowering in the bottle, is sweet and very pleasing when diluted or used in tiny amounts. Use it sparingly if you genuinely wish for contact with the angelic realm, or to come closer to your own angelic nature.

Benzoin
Styrax benzoin

Benzoin is a deep brown, thick, viscous substance with a smell reminiscent of vanilla. It relates very directly to the Base Chakra, on which it has a strongly energising effect. Use Benzoin when you need to increase physical strength and energy. At the same time, Benzoin is mentally calming and pacifying, especially useful for dispelling anger. If we consider that it is virtually impossible to offer healing, meditate or indeed do anything of spiritual value, while experiencing anger, Benzoin is truly a valuable aid.

Bergamot
Citrus bergamia

The green colour of Bergamot oil suggests an affinity with the Heart Chakra, and this is a particularly valuable oil where the Heart Chakra is affected by grief. When experiencing grief many people close the Heart Chakra making them unable to give or receive love and the uplifting, calming and joyous effect of Bergamot oil can assist in healing and reopening this centre once more to joy. Where the heart is already open, Bergamot can help an individual to radiate joy and healing to others.

Green is a calming colour and this oil can be used on any of the chakras if heat, disturbance or agitation is present.

Bergamot can be enhanced by using it in association with certain crystals.

CAUTION: Do not use undiluted on the skin before exposure to sunshine, as Bergamot increases the skin's sensitivity to the burning rays of the sun and severe burning can result. This effect lasts for quite a long time, so in sunny weather it is wiser to use Bergamot only on areas of the body that will not be exposed to the sun. Otherwise, restrict its use to burners, diffusers, etc.

Black Pepper
Piper nigra

Essential oil of Black Pepper is both a mental stimulant and a physical energiser. People who have a tendency to daydream or fall asleep during meditation (and that's all of us sometimes!) can benefit from using Black Pepper. Simply inhale the oil for a moment or two before sitting to meditate, or, indeed, at any other time when alertness and concentration are needed. Black Pepper also helps us to 'get a move on' at times when our lives feel 'stuck'. It helps move blocks that can prevent movement of energy between one chakra and another, especially between the Solar Plexus and Heart.

Camomile
Anthemis nobilis, Matricaria chamomila or Matricaria recutita

All Camomile oils share the same calming and soothing properties. These operate on all levels, physical, emotional and subtle. The deep blue colour of German Camomile (Matricaria varieties) indicates it affinity to the Throat Chakra, for which it is both strengthening and soothing. It is enhanced by using it in association with blue crystals such as blue Tourmaline.

Use it when there is a need for communication, for the truth to be spoken, but without anger or bitterness.

English Camomile (Anthemis Nobilis) is a paler, more ethereal blue in colour, which also relates to the Throat Chakra, but in its highest octaves. This oil can help individuals to express their highest spiritual truth, and may also assist channelling. Use it with paler blue gemstones (Blue Lace Agate or Aqua Aura, for example).

Blue is a calming colour generally, and Camomile can be used to counteract agitation or over-activity in any chakra. Use it also to heal the aura wherever heat, redness, anger, etc. are present.

Carrotseed
Daucus carota

Strengthens inner vision, enabling the user to perceive the highest truth at times of doubt or confusion. Helps to move blocks that prevent the free flow of energy, especially between the Solar Plexus and the Heart Chakra.

Cedarwood
Cedrus atlanticus

Cedarwood has been used as incense since time immemorial in civilisation as diverse Egypt and Tibet. It is still very actively used in Tibetan medicine and as a meditation aid by Tibetan Buddhists and others. It is thought to enhance spirituality and strengthen our connection with the Divine, and the wood was used in the construction of temples to symbolise this. It also helps us develop and maintain a sense of balance and control in our lives.

In physical applications Cedarwood is a powerful antiseptic and mucolytic (i.e. it breaks up catarrh) and we can see parallels in its subtle uses: helping us to cut through the 'mental catarrh' that can clog our minds just as surely as the physical variety clogs our noses.

The 'Cedar' which you may read of as being used by native American Indians in purification ceremonies ('smudging') is in fact a form of Juniper.

CAUTION: Cedarwood oil must not be used during pregnancy.

Clary Sage
Salvia sclarea

Clary Sage helps to bring us more closely in touch with the Dreamworld, which can teach us so many spiritual lessons. Clary seems to encourage vivid dreams, or it may be that it enhances dream recall. It may be used in evening baths, in a burner in the bedroom or a drop placed on the pillow. Before falling asleep focus on any problem or issue that needs clarification, with the conscious desire to receive help through dreaming. Keep a notebook near the bed to record any dreams on waking. Pay careful attention, too, to dreams that come unbidden, for they may throw light on issues of which you are not even aware at a conscious level. One of the old names for Clary Sage was 'Cleareye'. It was thought to strengthen the eyesight and the seeds of the herb (NOT the essential oil) were used to remove foreign bodies from the eyes. At the subtle level we may think of Clary as strengthening the inner eye and helping us to 'see' more clearly. Clary at the physical level is an aphrodisiac oil and this aspect may sometimes manifest as erotic dreams. These should not provoke guilt or any other negative feelings but simply tell us that some aspect of our sexuality needs clarifying.

CAUTION: Do not use Clary Sage during pregnancy. Do not use if you have taken any alcohol during the preceding few hours, or are likely to do so before long, as the combination of alcohol and Clary can lead to nightmares, rather than revealing dreams.

Cypress
Cupressus sempervirens

Cypress oil is helpful at times of transition such as career changes, moving home and major spiritual decisions such as changing one's religion. At such times the Bach Flower Remedy, Walnut can be used to great benefit as well. Cypress also helps with painful transitions such as bereavement or the ending of close relationships.

The Latin word 'sempervirens' in its name means 'ever-living' and refers to the evergreen leaves of the tree, but it may also be understood as referring to the afterlife, and both the ancient Romans and the Egyptians dedicated this tree to their gods of death and the afterworld. For thousands of years Cypress trees have been planted in cemeteries, perhaps as a reminder of the life everlasting and the essential oil can be used to give comfort and strength at the time of death, in the same way as Melissa.

Elemi
Canarium luzonicum

Elemi is distilled from the resin of a tree closely related to Frankincense and shares many of the same qualities. The aroma is also very similar. It has been used throughout the Arabic and Turkic world in ancient times. Its name, in Arabic means 'Above and Below', a contraction of 'As Above, so Below'. The oil has a unifying effect, helping to balance the upper and lower chakras, in somewhat the same way as Vetivert. It can also help us to balance our spiritual practices with our worldly responsibilities.

The balancing and unifying properties of Elemi are particularly valuable in group meditations, where it can help to bring the energies of all the participants into harmony quite quickly.

Elemi brings feelings of deep peacefulness combined with complete lucidity, which is especially helpful at the beginning of a period of meditation when it may not always be easy to shake off external preoccupations. It is helpful for all forms of meditation, but seems particularly to enhance visualization. Some people find that it makes them more open to mystical experiences. In this it resembles the action of Rosewood to some degree. At the end of a meditation it is of great value in enabling the mediator to return quickly to everyday reality even after very deep or prolonged meditation.

When used for chakra balancing in conjunction with certain crystals, Elemi may sometimes bring up deeply hidden emotions.

Eucalyptus
Eucalyptus globulus

Physically, Eucalyptus oil is a great antiseptic and purifier, burnt or vapourised in sickrooms to cleanse the air and speed recovery, and around the house during epidemics to help prevent the spread of infection.

Use it in the same way at a subtle level, to cleanse any place where there has been conflict such as rows and arguments, or even physical fighting, or anywhere where negative energies are felt.

Fennel
Foeniculum vulgare

Mediaeval herbalists describe Fennel as a protection against witches and evil spirits. If you feel threatened at any time by psychic attack, you might try burning or diffusing oil of Fennel, or rubbing a little of the essential oil on the Solar Plexus Chakra. Alternatively, rub a drop or two on your hands and smooth them over your aura at a little distance from the surface of the body.

Frankincense
Boswellia carteri

This oil is associated with the highest spiritual aspirations. It was offered to the infant Christ by the Magi in recognition of His divinity and it helps each of us to connect to that part of our selves which is eternal and divine.

Frankincense resin is one of the most ancient of the incenses, having been in use for at least 3,000 years and is also one of the most widely-used. The essential oil is both more powerful and more subtle in action because of the absence of solid matter. Unlike many of the oils used in subtle aromatherapy, we do make use of at least some of the physical properties of Frankincense particularly when using it as a meditation aid. Frankincense has the ability to deepen and slow the breath and this helps bring body and mind into a meditative state. This is valuable in ALL forms of meditation – not only awareness of the breath.

Frankincense helps break ties with the past, especially where these block personal growth. Use it in baths with the conscious intention of 'washing away' any old ties which feel like a hindrance, or in burners, perhaps combining this with the form of visualization suggested by Phyllis Krystal in 'Cutting the Ties that Bind'.

Helichrysum
Helichrysum italicum

These are the flowers, resembling a daisy or small chrysanthemum, which are sold dried by florists. For this reason the oil is sometimes sold under the French name 'Immortelle' and in America you will find it described as 'Everlasting'. I prefer to stick to the Latin to avoid confusion.

The oil has a sweet, honey-like aroma with a slightly bitter undertone. It is very strongly scented and can be quite overpowering when smelt from the bottle so it is particularly important with this oil to use it in the tiniest amounts only.

Its action is to activate the right (intuitive) side of the brain. This is of enormous value in all meditation, visualization, therapy and personal growth work as well as in the creative arts – music, painting, poetry, etc.

Helichrysum is said to induce feelings of compassion. I prefer to think that it puts us in touch with that part of ourself in which compassion flows freely. The oil mixes beautifully with Rose (use at least two drops of Rose to each drop of Helichrysum) to make a blend that unites the head and the heart.

Hyssop
Hyssopus officinalis

Hyssop has a very long history as a cleansing herb. It was used by both the Hebrews and the Egyptians to sweep out their temples and is mentioned several times in the Bible. You may like to use it to cleanse any area in which you are planning to meditate, give healing etc., though there are a number of cautions to be observed with this oil, and you may prefer to use one of the alternatives.

CAUTION: Do not use Hyssop during pregnancy, or if you suffer from high blood pressure or epilepsy – or if anybody likely to come into the area where you use the essential oil has any of these conditions.

Inula
Inula helenium

This oil is relatively little-used in conventional aromatherapy, having been introduced to the repertoire much later than many other oils. Its beautiful green colour immediately speaks of its affinity with the Heart Chakra. The effect is very strengthening, helpful to the 'faint-hearted' and to those who find it difficult to experience love or to express it. It is an important oil for those who are afraid to use their skills or gifts, or to allow the full beauty of their inner selves to shine out. The oil can be inhaled, used in massage or baths, or applied directly over the Heart Chakra.

Jasmine
Jasminium officinalis and Jasminium grandiflorum

Jasmine, more than any other oil, speaks to us of the unity of apparent opposites. Renowned for thousands of years as a powerful aphrodisiac, Jasmine is an equally potent aid to spiritual development. When Scott Cunningham writes 'When used with the appropriate visualization it can bring heightened spiritual awareness' he highlights what I have emphasised throughout this book: that the thought or intent of the user is a major factor in attuning to the subtle energies of the oils. He classifies Jasmine as a Yin oil, whereas Robert Tisserand calls it Yang – another manifestation of Jasmine's apparently paradoxical nature.

My own conclusion (based on intuition, meditation and dowsing) is that it is neither – or both. Jasmine brings together the strength and fiery dynamism we associate with Yang energy and the soft earthiness of Yin. As so often, contemplating the living plant leads us towards such knowledge. The delicate, almost fairy-like flowers are borne on a plant of great sturdiness and vigour. The creamy-white flowers yield an oil that is dark brown in colour and very deep in its aroma – without doubt a strong Base Note. But perhaps the most revealing fact is that Jasmine, unlike any other plant I know, is cared for by two Devas: a male and a female.

This is perhaps an indication of its most important application in Subtle Aromatherapy, the spiritualization of sexuality. With Jasmine we are helped to understand that there is no division between physical and Divine love. Rose and Neroli reveal other nuances of the same message – and it is interesting to consider for a moment that these three are so often bracketed together in traditional aromatherapy, too – but of the three Jasmine's message is the most powerful. In Marcel Lavabre's words 'It has the power to transcend physical love'.

Jasmine is thought to develop the artistic senses. For some people this may relate to their own creativity, for others it may make them more responsive to visual beauty, to music etc.

In common with Rose, this is an aroma favoured by the Angels. If you smell Jasmine when you know there is none nearby, an Angel has almost certainly passed your way. Conversely, if you wish to draw angelic beings towards you, use one drop of Jasmine with a suitable affirmation or visualization.

CAUTION: During pregnancy, this oil must not be used until birth is imminent, as it strengthens uterine contractions.

Juniper
Juniperus communis

Juniper oil has been used as a ritual incense for thousands of years and by civilisations as diverse as the Babylonians, Egyptians, Tibetans and Native Americans. It is a cleanser and detoxifier of both the physical body and the subtle bodies. It is particularly useful for clearing any negative energy that has accumulated, especially if this is through contact with other individuals with whom one does not feel in attunement. This may be applicable to such experiences as travel in public transport, to being in crowded places, being exposed to large numbers of people whom one does not necessarily know, or to contact with specific individuals, particularly if there has been anger, unpleasantness or ill-will expressed towards one's person, or unavoidable contact with people whose energies, actions or way of life are inimical to one's own spiritual path.

Ideally, Juniper can be used as a ritual bath in which case the cleansing power of water itself can be invoked as well as the cleansing power of Juniper. Very often, though, there may be a need for some cleansing before one is in a situation where physically bathing is possible. In this case it is quite simple to sprinkle one or two drops, not more, of Juniper oil on the palms of the hands and to stroke them light over the surface of the physical body, and/or over and through the aura. It is very important that in doing this, each stroke of the hands is taken right down to the ground, touching the earth and sweeping the negative energy away from the person needing to be cleansed. It is quite possible to cleanse oneself in this manner if there is nobody else available to do so. Just apply Juniper to both hands and stroke it over as much of the body as you can physically reach and move the hands through the aura at some distance from the body.

Juniper can also be used for cleansing rooms and buildings of any unwanted energy. This is particularly helpful when moving into a new house, or if some unpleasant event has taken place in your home. It is also helpful when conducting healing or meditation in a building that is not used all the time for such purposes. Simply put the oil in a burner or diffuser and allow the aroma to pervade the area that you wish to cleanse.

The American Indians burn dried sprigs of a form of Juniper (Juniperis virginiana) with other herbs in purification ceremonies, though confusion arises because this particular Juniper is usually referred to as Cedar in America.

Sometimes people feel a sense of uncleanliness in relation to their own lives. This may be due to past actions that they now regret or even to actions in previous lifetimes. It is possible to work with Juniper oil to help clear these feelings of uncleanliness from the most subtle layers of the aura. In this, Juniper's action resembles that of the Bach Flower Remedy Crab Apple, and some people may benefit by using both together.

CAUTION: Do not use in early pregnancy.

Lavender
Lavandula officinalis, or Lavandula vera

Lavender is known in traditional aromatherapy as the most versatile of oils: sedative, antiseptic, painkilling, antidepressant, calming and much more but, above all, balancing.

As so often, there are parallels between the physical and the subtle plane, and when used at the energetic level, Lavender is also calming, cleansing and balancing. The balancing action is seen particularly in relation to the Chakra system as Lavender helps to bring the higher and lower centres into harmony with each other. Like Vetivert, Lavender benefits all the chakras, with an action that is both calming and energizing. According to Philipe Mailhebiau it has a strong affinity for the Solar Plexus – again in common with Vetivert. (In fact, these two oils blend surprisingly well. Try using them together to enhance their action.) The action on the Solar Plexus helps to calm extremes of emotion.

The strongest affinity, though, is with the Crown Chakra or Thousand Petalled Lotus, where the expansive, healing nature of Lavender finds its fullest expression.

The calming, relaxing effects of Lavender can help in reaching deeper states of meditation, and those who channel while in trance may also find that this oil enables them to reach deeper levels of trance. This does not mean that everybody using Lavender is likely to go into a trance willy-nilly. Trance channelling is a gift given to very few. Once again, the oil works only with the user's intent.

Another balancing/harmonizing action of Lavender is in helping to integrate our spirituality into everyday life. Using Lavender can help us to know that our humblest actions are sacred.

Lavender oil is one of several that can be burnt or vapourised to cleanse a room or house of negative energies.

Mandarin
Citrus reticulata

Mandarin has many of the qualities of the other citrus oils, at both the physical and the subtle levels, but in a more refined and delicate form. Its delicate aroma breathes a message of happiness, especially to children and the child that is within each of us. It helps us to get in touch with that inner child. In its highest vibrations Mandarin embodies the energy of the Christchild.

Marjoram
Origanum majorana

Marjoram is associated with celibacy and can be of great help to anybody living a celibate life whether by choice, such as members of the priesthood or monastic orders of many different religions, or through force of circumstance, such as bereavement or temporary separation from a partner. Some people who are normally sexually active may also choose to remain celibate for specific periods of time, such as when taking part in a meditation retreat or receiving teachings from a spiritual master.

Marjoram oil diminishes the desire for sexual contact: this is a specific physical effect of the oil, particularly if used in nightly baths. At an emotional level, Marjoram has a comforting and warming effect which eases loneliness and grief. This particularly valuable when a loved partner has died.

CAUTION: Unless committed to lifelong celibacy, do not use Marjoram oil for lengthy periods of time, as it can eventually inhibit normal response. Prolonged use also has a deadening effect on the emotions. This oil should not be used during pregnancy.

Melissa
Melissa officinalis

Melissa oil, from the familiar garden Lemon Balm, has a very special place in subtle aromatherapy for its value at the time of death. It has long been known for its ability to bring comfort to the bereaved especially where a dear one has died suddenly, such as in an accident, so there is an element of shock, as well as grief. I have also found Melissa a great help and comfort to those who know that they are dying, as well as their friends and relatives. Its sweet, fresh fragrance seems to dispel fear and regret and bring acceptance and understanding as the time of death approaches. Used in a burner or diffuser in the dying person's room, this oil creates a feeling of spiritual unity that makes the approaching physical separation easier to accept.

Melissa has an affinity with both the Solar Plexus and Heart Chakras (its Swedish name means 'Heart's Joy') helping us to align our will with the Divine will and to expand our feelings of love from the individual and personal towards the total acceptance of unconditional love.

Melissa helps us to remember past lives. For some people it may facilitate past-life recall, while for others it instills or strengthens the understanding that they have lived before, even if they could not express that belief in words. Perhaps this is part of its value at the approach of death: by reminding us that we have lived before it also gives us the assurance that we can live again. The nature of the plant itself is symbolic of this. It is almost impossible to kill: even if cut back right to the ground it regenerates and quickly produces a mass of new growth.

The sense of spiritual unity referred to above, also makes Melissa useful for group meditation, especially where the group energy needs to be directed towards a common purpose.

SPECIAL NOTE: True oil of Melissa is very expensive, and other oils of similar smell, such as Lemongrass and Lemon Verbena are often substituted for it. These oils have their own properties, which are perfectly valid but are not the same as those of Melissa, so it is important to buy only from reputable suppliers who can guarantee that the oil is the one you are seeking. If it does not cost as much as Rose or Jasmine, it is certainly not Melissa.

Mugwort
Artemisia vulgaris

Various species of the Mugwort (Artemisia) family are used

213

in purification ceremonies by native American Indians, either alone or with other herbs, to purify places and people. The dried plants, usually bound together in a bundle known as a 'smudge stick' are burnt to produce a smoke, and the ceremony is known as smudging. Confusion may occur because several different varieties of Mugwort are known in America as Sage or Wild Sage, although they belong to a completely different botanical family. (This is another illustration of why it is so important to use the Latin names when buying oils.)

In Mediaeval and Renaissance Europe, Mugwort was hung up in houses to protect the occupants from evil.

CAUTION: Although the dried herb can safely be used in the ways described above, the essential oil of Mugwort is a hazardous one, and must NEVER be used during pregnancy.

Myrrh
Commiphora myrrha

Myrrh is one of the most renowned incenses along with its close relative, Frankincense and its known use goes back at least 4,000 years. Both were highly prized throughout the ancient world for their medicinal properties and their religious significance. Myrrh is thought to enhance and strengthen spirituality.

Use it as a meditation aid and before any healing session, either in burners or by inhaling directly.

Myrrh is a deep reddish-brown in colour, with a warming and stimulating effect on the physical body, and can be used to strengthen the Base Chakra when needed. Myrrh is particularly valuable for people who feel 'stuck' emotionally or spiritually and want to move forward in their lives.

CAUTION: Do not use during pregnancy.

Neroli
Citrus aurantium bigarada

Oil of Neroli, derived from orange-blossom, is associated with purity, perhaps because of the symbolism of the pure white flowers. Of the three oils which the orange tree yields, that from the flowers relates most closely to the spiritual life. When we are most immersed in worldly preoccupations, inhaling the bitter-sweet aroma of Neroli brings us in touch with our higher selves. Perhaps this is why it has such a profoundly calming and de-stressing action on the physical body as well as the mind.

Use Neroli in ritual baths for purification, in a burner to purify the place in which meditation or healing is to take place or inhale from a tissue to calm or to re-connect with the higher self.

Neroli has an affinity with the Eighth Chakra, and facilitates all spiritual work. It is also thought by some to enhance creativity, especially in relation to music and writing.

Neroli's reputation as an aphrodisiac is not as contradictory as it may at first appear. The ancient custom of crowning brides with a wreath of orange-blossom had the dual effect of symbolising virginity and allaying a young bride's possible anxiety about the wedding night. The ability of Neroli to help us connect with our higher self can serve to spiritualize sexual partnerships, bringing body and soul into union. To this end both partners should anoint the body with a single drop of the oil dissolved in 5 mls of almond oil or inhale one drop from a tissue, at the same time visualizing the union of their higher selves. Alternatively, each can take a ritual bath with three drops of Neroli while holding the same visualization.

Orange
Citrus aurantium

With Neroli (extracted from orange blossom) and Petitgrain (from the leaves), Orange oil from the rind of the fruit completes the trio of oils from the Orange tree. What generosity of spirit this tree exhibits: no other plant offers us three different essential oils. In comparison with the other two, this is a relatively simple oil in its character and actions, and it is interesting to note that it is, technically, not an essential oil but an essence as it is extracted from the orange rind by simple pressure, without the need for the complicated processes of distillation or enfleurage.

Its simplicity is its virtue – why create complication where none is needed?

Just as the fruit nourishes the body, the oil nourishes the soul, feeding it with feelings of joy. Use this oil when you feel joyous and experience its affinity with your own happiness. Use it, too, when you are sad, and be nourished by it. Use it to replenish anybody you know who is in need of cheer, and burn or vapourise it in any room or house if you feel that a more cheerful atmosphere needs to brought in.

Palmarosa
Cymbopogon martinii

The clean, flower-like scent of Palmarosa is thought to aid healing, so it is appropriate to use in areas where healing is offered. Use the oil in burners or diffusers in the room before a healing session. For absent healing, inhale a single drop of Palmarosa from a tissue while visualizing the person to be healed or, where a group meets to give absent healing, use a little Palmarosa in a burner during the meeting. If you work with crystals, you might like to place a single drop of the oil on a quartz crystal in the healing room when you are working.

Patchouli
Pogostemon patchouli

Patchouli oil is a deep brown in colour, sometimes with a reddish tinge, with a very deep, earthy aroma. In perfumery terms it is considered a Bass Note and at a subtle level the same holds true. The oil is associated with the Base Chakra, on which it exerts a strengthening and grounding effect. It also affects the second chakra, being considered by many authorities as an aphrodisiac. The second chakra is also associated with the watery elements of the body and Patchouli helps to reduce fluid retention in the physical body.

Patchouli is especially valuable for 'dreamers' and people who tend to neglect or feel detached from their physical bodies. This is a little trap into which many who are engaged on a spiritual path can fall, placing perhaps an undue share of importance on their mental/psychic experiences, to the detriment of their physical wellbeing. Patchouli helps to ground and integrate energy and keep us in touch with our physical selves.

It is as well to use this oil in the tiniest amounts only. Some people find the aroma quite unpleasant and this will negate any good effects it may otherwise have. It may be more effective used in a blend in minute proportions.

Peppermint
Mentha piperata

Peppermint acts upon the ego, dispelling pride. It helps equally to overcome feelings of inferiority – not as strange as it may seem, since undue pride often masks an inferiority complex. It is associated with cleanliness, and helps people who want to live an ethical life.

Petitgrain
Citrus aurantium (leaves)

Petitgrain oil is derived from the leaves of the orange tree, and therefore closely related to Neroli. There is some similarity in the aromas of the two oils, though Petitgrain is sharper. However, where Neroli evokes the highest psychic or spiritual levels of mind, Petitgrain relates more to the conscious, intellectual mind. Inhale this oil when you need mental clarity.

Pine
Pinus sylvestris

Pine oil is cleansing and invigorating, promoting feelings of energy and wellbeing and this is just as true at a subtle level as at the physical. It speeds healing of the physical body, though this oil is more appropriate for use in the actual presence of the ailing person rather than for absent healing – choose other oils for that purpose. Pine is good used in baths and especially in burners and diffusers. Use it to clear your healing or meditation space, especially if you are not able to devote a room exclusively to these uses and it is used for other purposes betweentimes. Bath in Pine sometimes as an alternative to Juniper when you have been in crowded places, public transport, etc.

Rose
Rosa centifolia, Rosa damascena, Rosa officinalis

Rose is, above all, the flower of love, both human and Divine. To the ancient Greeks, the Rose was the flower of Aphrodite, the goddess of love, beauty, the arts and creativity of all kinds. Aphrodite is better known to us now by her Roman name, Venus, and often thought of as personifying sensuality, though if you are familiar with astrology, you will know that the planet Venus is connected with the love of beauty in all its forms, including the arts.

To early Christian mystics, the Rose was the flower of the Virgin Mary. It still held the connotation of love, but in this context it symbolized Divine love and the union of Mary with the Holy Ghost. Both these symbolic uses of the Rose occur frequently in painting. Artists from the anonymous mediaeval masters to Velasquez show the Virgin crowned with Roses. Botticelli, the most mystical of Renaissance artists, depicts the goddess rising from the sea amid a shower of Roses in his 'Birth of Venus' and elsewhere paints the Madonna and

Child in a garden full of Roses. In this one flower the archetypes of Madonna and Whore are brought together and this tells us much about the subtle energy of Rose oil.

Rose is the supreme oil of the Heart Chakra, the centre of love, whether that be love for one person or Universal Love. The unfolding of a Rose, from bud to flower, symbolises the unfolding of love within the heart. It brings healing to the Heart Chakra and helps it to open again when grief has caused it to close down but where the chakra is already open, Rose strengthens its energy, enabling love energy to radiate out. It can also deepen the devotional expression of love for a Deity.

Rose has an equal affinity with the Sacral Chakra, the centre of creativity, sex and conception. It is a gentle aphrodisiac, and facilitates creativity in all the arts, but above all, by uniting within itself the human and the Divine aspects of love, Rose helps to spiritualise sexual relationships. The highest vibrations of Rose resonate with the Crown Chakra, the seat of the Guru Within.

Finally, do you know that Rose is the favourite perfume of Angels? If you wish to encourage Angels to enter your space, place bowls of fresh Roses there whenever you can, and spare a drop of your precious Rose Absolute to delight them and if you ever smell the delicate aroma of Rose when you know for certain that there are neither flowers nor oil anywhere near, you will know that an Angel has passed by.

Rosemary
Rosmarinus officinalis

Rosemary oil is a psychic protector, and as such it is particularly useful to use first thing in the morning before exposing oneself to all the external influences, both those of which we may be aware and possibly fearful and those of which we are not aware but may encounter in daily life. It is particularly appropriate to use Rosemary in the morning because at a physical level it is a stimulant and to use this oil later in the day may result in sleeplessness.

The oil can also be used for protection in houses, etc. Use it in a burner or vapouriser. This is one of the plants that was used in mediaeval Europe to drive out evil spirits from places or persons. Dried sprigs of the herb were burnt, and you might like to use it in this way as an alternative to the essential oil.

In relation to the chakras, Rosemary is particularly relevant to the Brow Chakra. In physical aromatherapy it is known as a cephalic oil, in other words, one which stimulates the brain and mental activity. At a subtle level Rosemary is associated with qualities of clear thought and clear-sightedness, and may be helpful wherever there is a need for clarity. At the most subtle level it may help the development of clairvoyance.

CAUTION: This oil must not be used by anybody suffering from epilepsy or high blood pressure. It should not be used late in the day as it will cause sleeplessness. Do not use during pregnancy.

Rosewood
Aniba roseodora

Rosewood oil is particularly associated with the Crown Chakra, and in the right circumstances can have an opening effect on this chakra. It is important to note that this will only take place if the person concerned is ready for this to happen. It would also appear that the action of this oil is very much dependent on the intent of those using it. When it is used casually, or for its physical effects, Rosewood appears not to affect the Crown Chakra of the user.

This is a particularly valuable oil to use for meditation or as a preparation for healing or any spiritual work. It also has an overall calming effect but without inducing any kind of drowsiness and this again can be very useful for meditation. Rosewood is also a subtle but real aphrodisiac.

Rosewood oil is distilled from a tree that is native to the Amazon rainforest, though most oil now available comes from sustainable plantations near the Brazillian coast. Ask about the origin of any oil you buy and use it only when genuinely needed, to avoid contributing to the destruction of the rainforest. Use Rosewood oil in meditations for the healing of the forests and of our beautiful planet as a whole.

NOTE: Ho-wood oil is NOT a substitute for Rosewood, and is potentially hazardous.

Sage
Salvia officinalis

The herb Sage has long been thought to promote wisdom. Whether this idea derives from the meaning of the word Sage – a wise man – or whether the herb was thus named because it was already thought to hold such properties is impossible to know. The Latin name, Salvia, denotes salvation, though this probably referred to salvation from physical illness. You might like to use Sage in conjunction with meditations or visualization to develop wisdom.

CAUTION: Sage is a hazardous oil, and should never be used by pregnant women, people suffering from epilepsy or other vulnerable groups. It is far safer to use the fresh leaves if you have access to a garden.

Sandalwood
Santalum album

Sandalwood has been used as an incense and meditational aid for thousands of years, the use originating in India where the trees are indigenous. Its particular value is that it quietens the mental chatter that can so often distract the meditator. By stilling the conscious mind, it allows the mind to move into the deepest states of meditation. This is also valuable in preparing for any healing work, and in self-healing. Visualization is also easier when the conscious mind can be temporarily put aside.

The odour is deep and extremely long-lasting and the oil is very thick and heavy in consistency. These properties suggest an affinity with the Base Chakra, which does in fact exist, but this oil also works at the level of the Crown Chakra in facilitating spiritual development. Sandalwood has connections with the Heart and Throat Chakras, and the aphrodisiac properties of the oil, which are very prominent, point to activity at the Sacral Chakra level. Sandalwood affects Chakra energy in so many different ways because it is a very complex oil, with many different actions at the subtle level. One of its greatest virtues lies in linking the Base with the Crown Chakra.

Spikenard
Nardostachys jatamansi

Spikenard (also known as Nard) intensifies feelings of devotion towards the Deity or towards a spiritual teacher. It embodies the spirit of generosity. These two emotions together with her pain at the knowledge of his imminent death led Mary Magdalene to anoint Jesus with Spikenard. It is a particularly comforting oil for people who work for Third World charities or aid agencies, and for those who experience deep inner pain over the suffering caused by natural and man-made disasters.

Thyme
Thymus vulgaris

Thyme oil is strengthening and energising at every level of being: physical, mental, emotional, etc. However, according to Scott Cunningham Thyme has the effect of closing down the psychic mind in favour of the conscious, intellectual mind. It might be helpful to bear this in mind and use Thyme only when conscious thought is needed, as opposed to spiritual intuitive or psychic effort. This particular effect of Thyme can help people who tend to be dreamy, detached or immersed in their spiritual life to the detriment of their mundane day-to-day functioning, also for anybody returning to work after a long retreat or a period of teaching from a spiritual master. At such times it can be very difficult to switch back into the everyday routine. A few drops of Thyme in the morning bath, or simply inhaling a drop from a tissue will help.

CAUTION: Thyme can be a rather aggressive oil. Pregnant women and other vulnerable groups should not use it, and a few drops in the bath really does mean a FEW unless you can obtain one of the gentle chemotypes of Thyme, such as Thymus vulgaris CT Linalol.

Vetivert
Vetiveria zizanoides

Vetivert is extracted from the roots of an aromatic grass, and is a deep brown oil with a somewhat viscous texture. All of these aspects suggest, quite correctly, a valuable grounding and earthing agent. Vetivert is very useful for anybody who needs to be brought into closer contact with the earth, to ground and centre their energies. For this the oil can be used in any of the methods described in this book. It also has a very special relationship with the chakra system, both generally and specifically. At a general level Vetivert is balancing to the chakra system, bringing the energies of all the major chakras into harmony, balance and alignment with each other. More specifically, it relates to the root chakra, as its colour, texture, aroma and origin in a root would suggest. For the root chakra Vetivert is calming and grounding, as opposed to an energising oil. However, possibly the most important use of Vetivert in relation to the chakra system is on the Solar Plexus Chakra to act as a protection against oversensitivity.

This oil applied to the Solar Plexus prevents one taking on too much of other people's 'junk', becoming a 'psychic sponge'. This protection may be obtained by applying Vetivert physically to the solar plexus area of the body, putting a single drop on the fingertips and gently applying it to the solar plexus in an anticlockwise circular direction. Or it may be used in the same way but making the anticlockwise circle some distance from the body – the method of use will depend entirely on the preference of the person using it. If they feel more reassured by physical application, then this is ideal. If the user is very sensitive to subtle energy and wishes to use the Vetivert within their aura, then this is alright too.

The balancing effects of Vetivert are valuable in group meditations, when used in a burner or diffuser, since it not only aligns individual energies, but can be used to balance and align the energies of all the people taking part in a meditation. Its grounding and earthing qualities are also important here, because it is vital for meditators to be able to return to life in the physical world and their daily activities at the end of their periods of meditation.

Some people find the deep, earthy scent of Vetivert an aphrodisiac. Its balancing nature reminds us that wholeness embraces both our physical and our spiritual selves.

Ylang Ylang
Cananga odorata

This very sweet oil helps to create a feeling of peace and dispel anger which is a hindrance to meditation, healing and all spiritual activities. However, Ylang Ylang is also a very soporific oil, so it is not recommended to use it immediately before sitting to meditate. Some people find its sweetness excessive and cloying, so it is often better to use it in a blend with Bergamot or Melissa which will enhance its pacifying powers as well as improving the aroma.

CHAPTER 17

Beyond the Essence

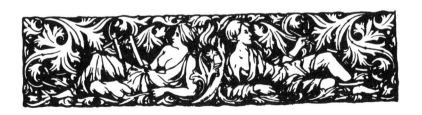

When we use essential oils, whether for physical aroma-therapy or in more subtle ways, it is easy to forget their origins within living plants, but if we want to appreciate and experience the healing powers and subtle energies of plants to the full, it is important to look beyond our little brown bottles.

Never forget the living plants, in all their wonderful diversity, which bless us with the gift of these precious oils. An essential oil is a summing-up of the qualities of a plant, it stands as a representative of that plant, but it can never entirely replace the beauty and power of that plant when it was whole and growing. It is as if in concentrating the perfume of the plant, we sacrifice its visible beauty and in doing so we lose some of the ways of knowing that plant and its energies at a deep, intuitive level. So it helps our understanding and sensitivity to come close to living plants as often as possible.

When you consider the growing plant, here are some of the things you might ask yourself:

What does it colour tell me? Is it soft and subtle, or vibrant and glowing? Look at the colour of leaves, stems, flowers and maybe fruit and bear in mind which part yields the essential oil. What does this suggest about the plant's energy and areas of healing?

What shape are the flowers? Are they simple or compli-cated, open and expansive in appearance or secretive and containing some mystery in their shape? What shape are the leaves? Are they simple or complicated? How do they relate to the flowers? Do they offset the flowers or hide them? Are their shapes similar or complementary? What can I learn from looking at these shapes?

What is its habit of growth? Is it tall and straight, or does it hug the earth? Is it fragile in appearance or strong and rugged? Is it spiky or rounded, straggling or compact, and what can these aspects tell me about its energies?

What is its texture. Is it rough, smooth, hairy, thorny, leathery? Look at both stems and leaves – are they similar in texture or different? What can I learn about this plant from its texture?

Above all, every time you use an oil, try to carry a clear picture of the plant or flower in your mind. When you give healing, encourage the receiver to form a mental picture of the plant, too. Surround yourself with pictures of the plants – photographs, paintings, botanical drawings and look at them often. Whenever possible, look at the living plant itself.

To visualize the plant when using it for healing, meditation, etc., adds another dimension to the energy on which you can draw: indeed, I have been told by my guides that I need only visualize any plant in order to draw upon its healing powers. I have to confess, though, that my love of the essential oils and their perfumes is so deep and of such long standing that I cannot imagine working without them, and I always use the oil and the visualization together. All the same, that might be worth knowing if one needed a particular oil that was not immediately available.

To develop to the fullest your intuitive understanding of healing plants, it is a good practice to meditate in the presence of living plants. You may do this to enhance your regular meditation, or as a preparation for a healing session. If you have the appropriate plants available in your garden and the weather allows, it is very beautiful to meditate in the open air, close to the living plant. Or you may be able to bring container grown plants indoors into your usual meditation space, or the place in which you give healing. Just spend some time quietly sitting near the plant, be open to its energy, allow yourself to be aware of the plant's aura. Contemplate the beauty and special qualities that are unique to this plant and give thanks for its existence on Earth. Consider the ways in which this plant may help you, or other people and, if appropriate, invoke its aid in healing yourself or any other person. You might like to imagine the plant being assimilated into your body, or your aura and the plant's aura merging with each other.

Try to have growing plants always present in the places where you meditate or give healing. These may well not be the aromatics that have been the subject of this book, since few of them are happy to grow indoors for any length of time, but all green plants add their beauty, grace and energy to your work. Fresh flowers will do so too and have the valuable ability to absorb negative energy. I try always to have cut flowers in any room where I give healing in the knowledge that when they fade and I take them away, I am also taking away any negativity that may have been released in healing sessions.

Above all, every time you come to the end of a healing session, a meditation or whatever purpose for which you have drawn on the unique and precious qualities of plants, remember to thank your friends in the plant kingdom for their help.

Be aware, too, of the precious soil in which the plants grow: the soil that is part of Gaia, our living planet. In drawing their nourishment from the very body of the Earth Mother plants make that nourishment readily available to us, to use as food, medicine, perfume, building materials, fabrics. Life on Earth would not be possible in its present form without plants.

So here, to close, is a meditation on the living plant, which has brought me closer to these fragrant, healing miracles of creation, and which I now share with you.

MEDITATION ON THE LIVING PLANT

Sit close to the plant you have chosen to contemplate, if possible in the open where the plant is growing. Spend some time looking at the plant with loving care. Notice every detail of the plant: the shape of the plant as a whole, its colour, the way the leaves are placed on the stems, the shape of the leaves. Touch a leaf to feel its texture, rub it gently between your fingers so that you can experience its aroma. If the plant is in flower, look at the flowers, at their shape, their colour, how they unfold from the bud. Gently inhale the fragrance of the flowers. Bring your hands close to the plant and feel its energy field.

Now close your eyes and form a mental picture of the plant. Try to re-experience all the sensations of sight, smell, touch, etc. connected with that plant. (Don't worry if you cannot recreate all of them – some people find visualization difficult, and many more find it impossible to recall smell. Persevere, knowing that simply trying to do this brings you closer to the plant at a subtle level.)

Now feel that the plant is merging with yourself at the level of your heart. Experience in your heart the loving energy that radiates from the plant for the purpose of healing and if there is anything within your own heart that needs to be healed, allow the healing to take place.

Feel the plant expanding and gently filling your whole body with its loving energy. Become aware of any part of your body that is in need of healing, and allow the energy of the plant to suffuse that area with love so that a healing process can begin.

Now feel the plant expanding beyond your physical body into your aura. Feel that the plant's energy field is one with your own. If you wish to extend healing to others during this meditation, do so now, using the auras of yourself and the plant, which are now as one. If you do not have a healing intent at this moment, simply dwell in this feeling of oneness with the plant.

Now, sitting united with the plant, begin to experience your connection with Gaia. Imagine roots growing from your feet down into the Earth, feeling their way through the dark, moist, nourishing soil. Draw up nourishment through your roots into your body. Feel your roots growing deeper and deeper through the soil until they reach down into the very centre of the Earth, into the molten lake of transmuting fire. Allow any pain, tiredness, grief or negative energy that is with you to flow down your roots into the fire, where it can be transformed. Draw up a stream of gold through your roots to fill your entire being. Feel your body completely suffused with golden light, and stay with this feeling for as long as you wish.

Gradually return your attention to the plant that is the subject of your meditation, and once again see it in front of you with your inner eye. Offer thanks to the plant for its beauty and for its healing. When you feel ready, slowly open your eyes and see the living plant before you.

Bibliography and Further Reading

La Medecine Aromatique, Fabrice Bardeau; Lafont, 1976.

The Healing Herbs of Edward Bach, Julian and Martine Barnard; Bach Educational Programme, 1988.

The Complete Herbal, Nicholas Culpeper, 1651.

Magical Aromatherapy, Scott Cunningham; Llewellyn Publications, 1990.

Massage and Meditation, George Downing; Random House, Inc., 1974.

What We May Be, Piero Ferrucci; Crucible (Aquarian Press), 1982.

Vibrational Medicine, Richard Gerber, M.D.; Bear and Co., 1988.

Flower Essences and Vibrational Healing, Gurudas; Cassandra Press, 1983 (1989).

The Spiritual Properties of Herbs, Gurudas; Cassandra Press, 1988.

The Holistic Herbal, David Hoffman; The Findhorn Press, 1983.

Chakras, Harish Johari; Destiny Books, 1987.

Chinese Medicine: The Web That Has No Weaver, Ted Kaptchuk; Century Hutchinson, 1987.

Cutting the Ties that Bind, Phyllis Krystal; Element Books, 1982.

Aromatherapy Workbook, Marcel Lavabre; Healing Arts Press, 1990.

Healing into Life and Death, Stephen Levine; Gateway Books, 1989.

A Handbook of Angels, H.C. Moolenburgh; The C.W. Daniel Co. Ltd., 1988.

Healing with Crystals, J. Pawlik and P.L. Chase; Newcastle Publishing Co. Inc., 1988.

Healing with Gemstones, J. Pawlik and P.L. Chase; Newcastle Publishing Co. Inc., 1989.

Crystal Enlightenment, Katrina Raphael; Aurora (distr. in England by Airlift Book Co.), 1985

Crystal Healing, Katrina Raphael; Aurora (distr. in England by Airlift Book Co.), 1987.

The Crystalline Transmission, Katrina Raphael; Aurora (distr. in England by Airlift Book Co.), 1990.

Messengers of Light, Terry Lynn Taylor; H.J. Kramer Inc., 1990.

The Art of Aromatherapy, Robert Tisserand; The C.W. Daniel Co. Ltd., 1977.

The Symbolism of the Rose, Dylan Warren-Davies; In *Aromatherapy Quarterly*, No. 29, Summer, 1991.

Aromatherapy: An A–Z, Patricia Davis; The C. W. Daniel Co. Ltd., 1988.

Appendix –
Useful Addresses

1. TUITION IN RELATED SUBJECTS

Aromatherapy

London School of Aromatherapy,
Swanfleet Centre, 93 Fortess Road,
LONDON NW5 1AG.

Write with s.a.e. for Prospectus of courses designed by Patricia Davis, ranging from one-day introductory seminars to full practitioner training, also Subtle Aromatherapy seminars.

International Federation of Aromatherapists,
Stamford House,
2/4 Chiswick High Road,
LONDON W4 1TH.

Have a list of affiliated schools (enclose s.a.e.).

Crystals

Opie Gems,
57 East Street,
ILMINSTER,
Somerset TA19 0AW

Flower essences

Clare Harvey,
Middle Picadilly, Holwell,
SHERBORNE, Dorset DT9 5LW.

Offers courses covering all the Flower Essences and Gem Elixirs.

Healing skills

David Cousins,
26 Pennsylvania,
LLANEDERYN, CARDIFF,
S. Wales CF3 7LN.

Workshops to develop spiritual awareness and healing ability.

2. SUPPLIERS OF MATERIALS MENTIONED IN THE TEXT

Essential oils

Aroma Vera Inc., 3384 So. Robertson Place,
LOS ANGELES, CA 90034, U.S.A.

Ask for their organic (biological) list.

Swanfleet Organics, Swanfleet Centre,
93 Fortess Road, LONDON NW5 1AG.

A range of organic and wild grown oils.

Fragrant Earth, P.O. BOX 182, TAUNTON, Somerset TA1 3SD.

Sell only organically produced or wild-grown oils.

N. and G. Rich, 2 Coval Gardens, LONDON SW14 7DG.

Have a small but growing range of organics.

Leydet Aromatics, P.O. BOX 2354, FAIR OAKS, CA 95628, U.S.A.

Essential oils, diffusers, etc.

Crystals

Earth Design Ltd, The Craft Centre, Broadwindsor,
BEAMINSTER, Dorset DT8 3PX.

Crystals, gemstones and minerals.

Opie Gems, 57 East Street, ILLMINSTER, Somerset TA19 0AW.

Crystals, gemstones, books, also Native American artefacts.

Chakra charts

Healing Art, P.O. Box 16, TOTNES, Devon TQ9 5UY

Full-colour posters designed by Patricia Davis showing the chakras with related essential oils and crystals. Also other aromatherapy charts, cards, etc.

Diffusers

Aroma Vera Inc.
Fragrant Earth
Leydet Aromatics
Swanfleet Organics

The addresses of all these suppliers are listed under ESSENTIAL OILS

Flower essences/flower remedies

The Alaskan Flower Essences, 1153 Donna Drive,
FAIRBANKS, Alaska 99712, U.S.A.

Flower and Environmental Essences.

236

Crystal Herbs, Waveney Lodge,
HOXNE, Suffolk IP21 4AS
The full range of 38 Flower Remedies, also Angel Essences and
Chakra Essences.

Crystal World, Anubis House, Creswell Drive,
RAVENSTONE, Leics LE6 2AG.
English distributors of Californian and Gurudas Flower Essences
and Gem Elixirs.

(There is, as yet, no English distributor for the Arizona, or Virginia
essences. You will need to write to the American addresses listed.)

Harebell Remedies, Monybuie, Corsock,
CASTLE DOUGLAS, Kirkudbrightshire DG7 2DY.
A range of newly-developed flower essences.

Healing Herbs Ltd., P.O. BOX 65, HEREFORD HR2 0UW.
The full range of Flower Remedies.

Haakon and Melinda Lovell, Bright Star, 90 Eebury Road,
RICKMANSWORTH, Herts WD3 2BH.
Sets of 36 gem essences, environmental essences and newly-
developed Essences of Our Lady which combine flowers and gems.

Pegasus Products Inc., P.O. BOX 228, BOULDER,
CO 80306, U.S.A.
California Flower Essences and Gem Elixirs.

Perelandra Ltd., BOX 136, JEFFERSONSTOWN,
VA 22724, U.S.A.
All the Virginian Flower Essences, Rose and Garden Essences.

Shambala, Coursing Batch, GLASTONBURY,
Somerset BA6 8BH.
English suppliers of the Alaskan Flower Essences.

Smudging herbs and incenses

Star Child, The Courtyard, 2-4 High Street,
GLASTONBURY, Somerset BA6 9DU.
A range of excellent incenses.

Twinlight Trail, 2 Buckingham Lodge, Muswell Hill,
LONDON N10 3TG.
Smudging herbs and incenses.

Raditech

Dulwich Health Society, 130 Gipsy Hill, LONDON SE19 1PL.
Suppliers of RadiTech, MagniTech, books and Pamphlets about
geopathic stress. Consultations with Dowsers and contact with
local dowsers.

3. PROFESSIONAL ASSOCIATIONS

American AromaTherapy Association,
P.O. BOX 3679, SOUTH PASADENA, CA 91031, U.S.A.

International Federation of Aromatherapists,
Stamford House, 2/4 Chiswick High Road,
LONDON W4 1TH.

National Association for Holistic Aromatherapy,
P.O. BOX 17622, BOULDER, CO 80308-7622, U.S.A.

4. OTHER USEFUL ADDRESSES

Aromatherapy-in-Care,
c/o International Federation of Aromatherapists
(address above).

A network of aromatherapists working in hospitals and hospices.
Provides peer support. (I.F.A. Full Members only.)

Aura Vision, Schmied-Kochel-Str. 22,
D-800 MUNCHEN 70, Germany.

and

Aura Vision, 28308 Seminary Avenue, OAKLAND,
CA 94605, U.S.A.

For photographs of the human aura.

Cruse, 126 Sheen Road, RICHMOND, Surrey TW9 1UR.

Bereavement counselling and other support. Send s.a.e. for local contacts.

Fountain International, P.O. BOX 552, TORQUAY,
Devon TQ2 8PE.

Environment Healing Network. Send s.a.e. for details of your nearest group.

The Institute of Building Biology, White Horse House, ASHDON,
SAFFRON WALDEN, Essex.

Promotes environmentally-conscious building, combining care for the environment and health factors in buildings. Can provide information, pictures and consultations.

Kirlian Institute, 173 Woburn Towers, Broomcroft Avenue,
NORTHOLT UB5 6HU.

Information about Kirlian Photography, including medical use, data on all the various uses on record.

Index